About the

Sophie Boss and Audrey Boss are sisters and co-founders of Beyond Chocolate, offering women a radically new approach to weight-loss and body confidence. They are on a mission to empower women to trust their bodies and free themselves from the shackles of dieting and overeating. Sophie and Audrey live with their families in North London.

For more information, visit www.beyondchocolate.co.uk.

Beyond
Temptation

How to stop overeating and feel normal and in control around food

Sophie Boss and Audrey Boss

piatkus

PIATKUS

First published in Great Britain in 2012 by Piatkus
This paperback edition published in 2013 by Piatkus

A CIP catalogue record for this book
is available from the British Library.

ISBN 978-0-7499-5736-0

Design and typesetting by Paul Saunders
Illustrations by Sabrina Oliva
Printed and bound in Great Britain by
Clays Ltd, St Ives plc

Papers used by Piatkus are from well-managed forests
and other responsible sources.

MIX
Paper from
responsible sources
FSC® C104740

Piatkus
An imprint of
Little, Brown Book Group
100 Victoria Embankment
London EC4Y ODY

An Hachette UK Company
www.hachette.co.uk
www.piatkus.co.uk

For

Alice, Becky, Christine, Debbie, Emily, Fatima,
Grace, Heather, Isabelle, Jane, Kate, Leila, Natasha,
Olivia and Pam.
Whoever you are, wherever you are.

Contents

Go!   141

Acknowledgements

IT TAKES MORE THAN an author (or two) to write a book. Literally thousands of people have contributed to *Beyond Temptation*. A huge thank you to all the women who have shared their stories with us over the years with courage and honesty. This book would simply not have been written without the Beyond Chocolate community. And it would not have been published without the support of all those at Piatkus who believed in this project from the very beginning. Special thanks to Zoe Goodkin our editor whose insightful feedback helped us shape this book every step of the way.

Sabrina Oliva's illustrations have brought the *Beyond Temptation* process to life, way beyond our expectations. We are so glad she didn't listen to her own Gremlins; we knew she could do it.

One of the things we most enjoy about writing books is taking ourselves away from the madness of our busy lives to the sanctuary of beautiful, peaceful places where we can immerse ourselves in the work. A heartfelt thank you to Leonie and Paolo at La Rascina for creating the perfect space. We will be back for more, *grazie*. And while we are away, we can relax safe in the knowledge that our wonderful Fairy Clare is back at Beyond Chocolate HQ keeping everything tickety boo, running like clockwork. We couldn't do it without her.

Last, but obviously far from least, we are so grateful to our families who believe in us and all the work we do with Beyond Chocolate. Thank you a million times over to Johnny, who becomes the perfect house husband and looks after Oscar while Mummy goes away to write her chocolate books. Huge gratitude to Ben for his solid, unwavering support and to Jasper and Evie for their patience and understanding when it seems as if Mum has been swallowed up by her computer. And finally, we are so thankful to Manou for hopping on planes at a moment's notice to be the perfect grandmother.

Introduction

SOPHIE: I spent the best part of my life, from the age of twelve to thirty-four, either on a diet, desperately trying to lose weight or in between diets constantly overeating, obsessing about food all the time. For twenty-two years, I longed to feel normal and in control. I struggled with everything to do with food and eating, every single day. I overate, put on weight and felt bad about myself and my body. Overeating was my way of taking care of myself and punishing myself at the same time. Sounds irrational? I think my eating *was* irrational. It didn't make sense and yet it *did* work. It helped me to stuff down the things I didn't know how to talk about. Overeating allowed me to be the good girl on the outside, even though I was being the bad girl in secret. Food helped me to numb the emotions I wasn't comfortable with or didn't understand. It helped me to distract myself when I needed distracting and it filled the time when I didn't know what to do with myself.

Eating was my answer to pretty much everything. I'd eat, and then I'd beat myself up for being so weak and out of control. I would shame myself into yet another useless diet, which did sometimes lead to weight loss, but which never helped me change my destructive overeating patterns. In fact, the diets compounded and cemented them. Food was my best friend and my worst enemy, all rolled into one. I felt desperate, and when I didn't know where else to turn, there was *always* food.

I remember buying a pack of six lemon drizzle slices from Marks & Spencer. I told myself I'd eat just one with a cup of tea when I got home. Minutes later there I was sitting in the car, still in the car park, ripping open the pack. The first one tasted wonderful. That lemony zing, the sugary icing, the soft, springy sponge. And I just couldn't stop. I had another and then another and then another. Eating fast, feeling guilty. I stuffed in the last two, almost in tears, disgusted with myself. I just couldn't take them home. How would I explain where the others had gone?

I remember a few days later, another trip to M&S. This time a box of four cream-filled chocolate eclairs. In the car again. Eating them all. Feeling sick. Not really wanting the last one, stuffing it in almost as a punishment for being so weak and disgusting.

I remember clearing up after a dinner with friends when everyone had gone home. Alone in the kitchen. As I piled the plates into the dishwasher, I gorged myself on cold roast potatoes, congealed chicken and leftover crumble. On automatic pilot, not thinking, not feeling. Numb.

I remember a weekend on my own at home. Just me and the food. As I watched the film I'd rented, I ploughed my way through all the treats I'd stocked up on. In just an hour and a half I methodically devoured a large bag of Kettle Chips, a Kit Kat, three crumpets (dripping with butter), four slices of processed cheese, a pack of chocolate fingers, a bag of jumbo peanuts, a tube of fruit pastels, a chicken curry from Marks – alternating sweet and savoury. On and on. All evening. Not stopping for an instant.

I remember sitting down to a meal with Ben and the children. I'd made enough pasta to feed the four of us and the family next door! I ate one helping and then another and another. Feeling stuffed to bursting, desperate to keep eating, not wanting it to end.

I remember visiting my parents in Paris and going into town to do some shopping. The afternoon was punctuated with eating pitstops. A croissant and a pain au raisin from my favourite patisserie. Four macaroons from Ladurée. A piece of baguette with a bar of chocolate sandwiched inside (a throwback to my school days). A wedge of Camembert from the cheese shop, eaten on the go as I walked down the street. A tube of sweet chestnut purée, squeezed straight into my mouth. I ate constantly, all afternoon.

I remember when I was fifteen, sneaking out of my room really quietly to fill up a little bowl with peanuts over and over again, night after night. Terrified my mum would catch me and vowing each time that this was the last bowl.

I remember buying two French sticks for dinner and eating one with an entire packet of butter before anyone came home. Feeling sick and disgusted with myself as I picked at my dinner and the children fought over the bread, moaning I never bought enough.

I remember hiding under my duvet at boarding school, secretly, silently eating a packet of Monster Munch. Handling the packet so carefully to make sure it didn't rustle. Sucking each one slowly and carefully to make sure no one would hear, not daring to crunch. Terrified that I'd be discovered. Tense all over. Desperate to finish the pack, yet longing for the reassuring comfort to last all night.

I remember being exhausted at the end of the day, but for some reason not wanting to go to sleep. I would take a book to bed with a bowl of something to nibble – anything really. Ideally, crisps or nuts or salty snacks, but more often than not I didn't keep those foods in the house in a vain attempt to stop eating them, so I would make do with Ryvita or matzo spread with butter and Marmite. I ate and read, with regular trips back for more, propping my eyes open until I fell asleep in the crumbs, full and disgusted.

I remember going to the cinema with a friend and not being able to resist the large box of sweet popcorn. I lied and casually alluded to not having had time for dinner, too ashamed to admit that I was already full. Worrying that she would think I was greedy.

I remember revising for exams, giving myself a break by baking a Madeira and glacé cherry cake and then sitting down with a cup of tea and one large slice. And then another. And another. Tidying it up, so that there was just a half left. And then a quarter. Making it nice and neat.

I remember bingeing on free foods when I was doing Weight Watchers. Spending hours painstakingly working out how many points I had left and then filling myself up with carrot sticks, celery, gherkins, cherry tomatoes and Diet Coke.

I felt so out of control, so alone. There was no one I could talk to about it. How could I when I felt so ashamed and disgusted with myself? No one else could possibly be this hopeless; no one would understand. And I had no idea what to do about it.

Then, in 1998, thanks to Audrey, I came across a radical idea: that dieting was contributing to (or even the cause of) my overeating and weight gain and that the answer was to STOP dieting for good. For ever. Back then, it was unheard of, a completely revolutionary notion and a pretty scary thing to do. I had nothing to lose. So I stopped dieting. I threw away my scales. I dumped the diet books and the calorie counters. I cut up my Weight Watchers gold card. And I just stopped. It is the bravest decision I have ever made.

I have spent the twelve years since then exploring and working on every aspect on my relationship with food and my body. And because of the kind of woman I am, as soon as I realised how liberating and empowering it was to ditch the diets, I wanted to shout about it from the rooftops. I wanted to talk about it with other women, to offer them an alternative – something of real value. And, in so doing, I knew I would support myself and the changes I was making too.

So Audrey and I created Beyond Chocolate. We ran workshops, designed ecourses, wrote a book and worked with thousands of women. It was exciting and incredibly satisfying to see our participants walk away freed, literally, from the shackles of dieting.

Today, my relationship with food is relaxed and comfortable. I don't stress or worry about it. Looking back, I realise that I *was* normal then because, sadly, overeating and feeling out of control *is* the norm among women in our society. So today, I am one of the lucky few who has a healthy, balanced relationship with food and that is far from normal.

I eat foods that I like – foods that nourish me in lots of ways. I eat when I'm hungry and, most of the time, I stop when I've had enough, when my body is sated. I don't turn to food when I'm feeling upset or anxious or pissed off. These days, I know what to do with those feelings; I don't need to eat them away. Occasionally, I choose to eat more than my body needs – because I like the food, because it does the job I want it to do in the moment, because if I didn't eat cake just because I fancy it, I'd probably never eat cake! (When I'm hungry, it's just not what my body asks for.) And a life without cake (particularly Audrey's home-baked beauties) would not suit me one bit. I never feel bad or guilty if I overeat and I don't beat myself up about it.

I have stopped pushing myself into punitive and boring exercise plans. I move for enjoyment, for the joy of using my body and, as a result, I am fit and healthy. The way I eat works for me, and the body I have as a result does too. My body is what it is; it's not perfect and I like it just as it is.

Since we started Beyond Chocolate, I have worked with thousands of women who struggle with their eating, who hate their bodies, who overeat, who binge and purge, who think that they are hopeless cases and that nothing will ever work for them. Every session with clients, every workshop, every group, renews my commitment to empowering women to know and trust their bodies. Every woman I work with inspires me and fuels my determination to keep speaking out, to keep talking about what it's really like to struggle with the way we eat and the way we look: to expose the absurdity of the simplistic (and counterproductive) notion that all we need do is get a grip, eat less and move more.

AUDREY: I can't remember when I first came across the idea of purging to control my weight. I was certainly making myself throw up regularly by my early twenties and I had been playing around with it for years before that. By the time I reached my early thirties, I was vomiting up to three times a day. By then, I had had a calcified saliva gland surgically removed and was battling with ongoing gum disease as a result. And yet, until that moment, I'd never really seen my bulimia as a problem. Although I eventually had to admit that I was killing myself very slowly and that I needed to stop if I wanted to stay alive, it wasn't the vomiting that I felt so awful and out of control about. It was the overeating that went hand in hand with it – the overeating that I did just before . . . and sometimes just after I vomited. It was the overeating that I felt powerless to stop.

Overeating, bulimia, dieting, worrying about my weight, hating my body: all of this kept me very busy – busy with the logistics and busy dealing with the self-disgust and despair. I spent so much time and energy planning binges, making up diets and with my head stuck down the toilet that there was little time to think about the really intolerable stuff in my life.

Food was my escape. Like Sophie, I ate to escape feelings I didn't know how to cope with. I ate to smother fears, suffocate anger, stifle sadness and curb my enthusiasm. I ate to escape physical discomfort, the chocolate and sweets soothing like a massage. I ate to forget unhappy relationships, losing myself in the comfort of food. I ate to avoid myself, to keep myself busy. And the more I ate, the more I felt ashamed and weak and out of control.

I remember going to the posh patisserie down the road and buying a birthday cake, making a point of telling the owner that it was for my niece. I went home and ate the whole thing, feeling ashamed and disgusted with myself for being a liar *and* a pig.

I remember eating my way through bags and bags of licorice wheels, my teeth aching from the sugar, my gums sore, my tongue furry and my lips chapped, shovelling them in, without pause, just eating and eating and eating. I remember feeling the self-disgust even while eating, but the rest of me was caught up, unable to stop.

I remember, midway through a diet, sitting in my kitchen in the dark, late at night eating sheet after sheet of stale matzo with honey because that's all I had in the house. I ate and ate, pausing only to spread more honey on new sheets until it was all gone and I was left with nothing but sticky hands and despair: despair at how much I'd eaten, despair at failing yet another diet and being so out of control and despair at the thought of being fat for ever.

I remember buying a six-pack of low-fat yoghurts to last me the week and eating them all in one go, feeling sick and weak and pathetic as I spooned the goo into my mouth.

I remember staying over at a friend's house for the night and raiding their kitchen cupboards in the wee hours, eating anything that was already open or looked like it wouldn't be missed. I crept back to my bed, terrified they would find out and expose me for the fraud I was, tossing and turning in bed, feeling ill and ashamed.

I remember going out to an expensive restaurant with clients and making myself throw up in between courses, so I could justify eating the next one. I would make sure I filled my glass of water before I disappeared into the toilet so I could cleanse my mouth of the sour taste of vomit before starting to eat again.

I remember being at school and dashing to the toilets every now and again to hurriedly stuff myself with chocolate while sitting on the loo, pants around my ankles. Before going back to class, I would flush the toilet and pop a Tic Tac in my mouth, worried that people would smell the chocolate on my breath and find out how awful I was.

I remember going to dinner parties, pretending I was starving and sitting down to a three-course meal, having spent all afternoon bingeing at home beforehand. I would smile and talk and eat and laugh, feeling nauseous and wretched inside.

I remember buying my aunt a packet of lovely hand-made

biscuits to take back as a souvenir from a holiday and methodically eating my way through the entire pack on the train home berating myself for being so selfish and greedy.

I remember going to the corner shop and buying loads of sweets, pretending to the nice man behind the till that I was babysitting and asking him to put them in three separate little paper bags so 'Alex, Silvia and Jack' could have one each. My ears burned with shame and I couldn't look him in the eye as I handed over the money.

I remember eating a whole box of Bendicks Bittermints one evening, then getting up in the morning to dash to the supermarket and replace them before my boyfriend woke up and realised what a greedy pig I was.

I remember planning my binges on my way to work, spending all day making lists in my head, feeling excitement and dread at the same time. I would go out of my way to avoid the local shop, and I'd stock up: bags of Haribos, cashew nuts, crumpets, chocolate cake, salami, bread, cheese, olives, tinned peaches – anything that looked 'good'. I would walk home weighed down by the heavy bags and a heavy heart, already knowing that all the food in the world would not satisfy my craving for love and companionship.

Then, about thirteen years ago, I woke up one morning and decided to stop. I decided to take control and put an end to the vicious cycle of overeating, vomiting, shame and body hatred. For the past decade, I have been exploring my relationship with food and with my body from every angle. I have had therapy, I created Beyond Chocolate with Sophie, I went on women's workshops and retreats. I have sat with thousands of women, listening to their stories, showing them a way forward, guiding them to work out their own answers. I have read books, so many books and even ended up writing two.

I have come away from every one of these experiences with insights, tools, support and self-awareness, as well a sense of renewed commitment to myself and to all the women out there who are miserable about the way they eat and how they look.

Today, I feel balanced and in control around food. I have a host of tools that I can use to cope with the ups and downs of life. Bingeing and vomiting do not figure on the list. Do I ever overeat? Yes, occasionally. My mum's meatballs with peas and rice, very creamy cauliflower cheese, bacon and avocado sarnies, malt loaf spread thickly with butter and Licorice Allsorts . . . these are just a few of my favourite comfort foods. They are the ones I sometimes turn to when I've had a rough day, am in need of a pick-me-up, in the week before my period and when it's cold and grey outside. They are like old friends – I know they are there for me when I need them and that they can be relied on to provide the comfort I am looking for. The huge difference now is that these moments are the exception rather than the rule, and that guilt, remorse, secrecy and shame are not part of the experience. Food is no longer the enemy.

◆

In this book, we are going to share everything we have learned about how to stop overeating and feel normal and in control around food. There is no rulebook for how to have a balanced and healthy relationship with food. There is no blueprint, there are no absolutes. What excites us about the work we do with Beyond Chocolate and Beyond Temptation is that it is honest. We aren't promising magic fixes and immediate transformation. What we deliver, over and over again, and what you will find in this book, is the possibility of true nourishment and the opportunity to take charge and make decisions about what and how much to eat and when to stop. We give women the tools to discover how they want their relationship with food to be and we show them how to get it. There *is* an element of magic in that, because when we are willing to take a risk – to go beyond the superficial, beyond the diets and the weight loss – we don't only find the key to transforming our relationship with food, we transform our lives.

What lies Beyond Temptation is self-confidence, peace of mind and freedom.

CHAPTER ONE

•

Can We Tempt You?

YEARS AGO, WHEN WE imagined ourselves normal, we never imagined that normal would involve overeating. When we looked at the women around us who we wanted to be like, the ones who seemed 'normal', we saw women who looked like they ate very little and were, invariably, thin.

Over the years, we have come to realise that normality is very rare in the woman/food equation. We have met literally only a handful of women who have a naturally easy, balanced relationship with food and their bodies. We have worked with thin women who overeat and purge, thin women who overeat and starve themselves, thin women who overeat and exercise relentlessly, thin women who hate their bodies and thin women who feel completely out of control around food.

Being thin or slim is not an indicator of a healthy, balanced attitude to food or of good health in general. And yet weight loss is the primary goal of health professionals and diet companies, and it has been for years. They are not interested in guiding us to a healthy and balanced relationship with food and a healthy body; they just want us to lose weight. Billions of pounds have been invested by governments in funding local and national programmes based on the calories in/calories out and eat less/move more theories which have failed us miserably. Despite a growing movement for a change in policy, we continue to be offered weight loss as the solution to everything.

Thankfully more and more scientists, doctors, activists, academics and writers today are advocating a different approach: an approach that involves looking to the root of the problem, rather than focusing on the weight, which is only the symptom. More and more of us are speaking out against the diet madness and offering a new way forward.

It's time to stop looking to the *so-called* experts, the self-styled doctors, the media or celebrities for the answers.

WEIGHT LOSS IS NOT THE GOAL

If you are reading this book, the likelihood is that you are either overweight, think you are overweight or are desperate not to be.

Let's be clear, when we use the words overweight and fat, this could mean any size. If you *think* you're fat, then you will behave as if you are, whether you are a size 6, 16 or 26. Feeling fat has very little to do with our actual body size.

It's time to let go of the notion that a body size is the answer to our problems, to stop holding on to the dream that achieving our goal weight will make everything okay. When we stop pinning all our hopes on a body size or a target weight, we are faced with the reality that everything is not perfect in our lives and probably never will be. We are finally free to step out of stereotypes and labels. We can see ourselves as we truly are.

We have no idea what weight you'll be when you stop overeating because the goal of this book is not to help you lose weight. You *may* lose weight, you may put some on and you may stay exactly as you are today. It depends on how much you weigh now. It depends on how much you've dieted in the past and what those diets have done to your body. It depends on how old you are. It depends on the types of food you eat, your genes, your constitution and so much more. Put into practice the ideas in this book and we can guarantee you this: when you stop overeating you will be a happier, healthier, more balanced person. And that you can be at any size.

So, how *do* you stop overeating? Virtually every conventional approach deals with overeating in one of two ways.

The just-stop-it approach

The dieting industry's favourite answer to overeating is simply to tell you to STOP IT! You know it's bad for you. You know it's why you're overweight. You'll feel better if you don't. So just stop it. Summon every ounce of willpower or determination or whatever it takes to resist the urge and control yourself. If you want to lose weight badly enough, then you'll do it, right?

The overeat-but-only-on-free-foods approach

Some programmes incorporate overeating as part of their solution. The alternative to eating too many chocolate bars is to overeat as much as you like, as long as you choose foods that they say are not fattening. They suggest you turn to low-calorie, low-fat, low-carb foods (or whatever isn't on their 'forbidden' list) or fill yourself up with low-calorie drinks. Binge on carrot sticks or celery, stuff yourself with 'free' soup, cram in as much cucumber or spinach as you like, nibble on rice cakes all day, if it helps, or pick at lettuce leaves and sunflower seeds in an attempt to satiate the insatiable. Some of these programmes positively *encourage* overeating, with days when you can eat as much as you like as long as you stick to certain foods. They go as far as to exhort you to pile your plate with as much as you want.

✦

What neither of these approaches addresses is the question of *why* we overeat and how we can stop. Not just for a few weeks or months, but for good. Relying on willpower or simply replacing overeating chocolate with overeating carrots is not the answer. The sad reality is that the diets pave the way to overeating. Whatever diet we choose, we spend so much time depriving ourselves of the food we really want that as soon as we give up dieting, we're eating for Britain – overeating all those off-limits goodies and taking the brakes off . . . until the next diet.

THE BEYOND TEMPTATION APPROACH

In our first book *Beyond Chocolate – How to stop yo-yo dieting and lose weight for good* (2006), we wrote about our own experiences as women who had struggled with our weight for years. We shared our personal stories and described how we transformed our relationship with food and our bodies.

It's six years since we wrote *Beyond Chocolate* and we haven't stopped exploring and experimenting for a minute. We certainly have not stood still, happy in the knowledge that we've cracked it. The ten principles in that book are the basis of a healthy and balanced relationship with food; we didn't invent them (well, the 'Be your own guru' principle is unique to Beyond Chocolate) – we simply took age-old, commonsense ideas and made them accessible. And since then, we've been looking at overeating in depth, questioning, investigating and watching all our wonderful participants grappling and experimenting.

Out of their work and ours has emerged a process, a way of engaging with the part of us that is driven to overeat – the part that turns to food for comfort, or sweetness, or distraction, or pleasure or just because it's there; the part that falls into the same trap over and over again, despite our very best intentions, despite everything we know. The process we have created is not only unique and effective, it teaches us so much about ourselves and our overeating that we believe it enriches every part of our lives.

The aim of this book is to guide you to stop overeating and discover how to live your life without turning to food – any food – as a treat, a salve or an escape. The way to stop is to identify the reasons why you overeat and then deal with them, using a set of practical, effective tools.

We'll be taking you on an overeating tour and, by the end of it, you will have all the information, insights, experience and tools you need for a relationship with food which feels balanced, healthy and free.

How long will it take?

The one question we are asked over and over again is 'How long will it take – how long before I stop overeating?'

How long it will take depends on a whole host of things: on how long you've been overeating and how much you rely on it;

on how long you've been dieting and how hooked you are on the diet mentality; on the kind of person you are and the way you respond to making changes in your life; and on how willing you are to experiment with the ideas in this book.

It can take anything from a few months to a few years – it's very, very likely to take more than a few weeks. In some ways, the slower the better. We are so used to quick fixes, so attracted to speedy, easy, effortless change that embarking on a process which takes time, effort, patience, perseverance and active participation on our part can feel frustrating and painfully slow. It's worth it. Honestly. If you are willing to take your time and to resist the urge to take shortcuts, you will be making changes that are both profound and sustainable.

So however long it takes, stick with it and keep taking action. Whether you spend a week or a month on each chapter before moving on to the next one, make it as easy and do-able for yourself as you can and, dare we say it, you might even enjoy the process. We sincerely hope you do.

Before you begin to make any changes or experiment with doing something different, we will be inviting you to do nothing other than observe yourself and gather information. We encourage you to be curious about yourself, interested in what you do, how you do it and what that's like for you. The more you get to know about yourself and your relationship with food, the better equipped you will be to make changes when you're ready. Change too soon, without exploring and understanding how you use food, and you will most likely do nothing more than go through the motions, turning this book into a diet-like programme and creating a set of rules for yourself. Which is likely to end the way all diets do; with you spiralling back into overeating, thinking, *This didn't work either* and looking for the next magic wand.

Take your time. How long have you been using food as a way of dealing with the challenges of life? Years? Decades? This is a beginning. You are opening the door to new possibilities: to freedom and peace of mind, to a relationship with food that nourishes and sustains you and a relationship with yourself that is authentic and honest.

SO MANY WOMEN ...

Over the years, we have had the privilege of working with thousands of women whose stories have inspired us and fuelled our commitment and determination to keep writing, offering an alternative to useless and counterproductive diets.

All those women have a voice in this book. We have drawn on their stories to create a group of characters, all of them fictional, yet all of them so real. We've named each one with a different letter of the alphabet. We'd like you to meet: Alice, Becky, Christine, Debbie, Emily, Fatima, Grace, Heather, Isabelle, Jane, Kate, Leila, Natasha, Olivia and Pam. Ordinary women, like you, like us. Women who overeat and are desperate to find a way to stop.

They are not caricatures or *types*; we don't believe in labelling people or putting women in boxes. We are all different. The way we overeat, the reasons we do it, the kinds of food we turn to – no two women are exactly the same and yet we share a common experience and a universal shame for doing what we do.

We imagine that you may identify with parts of several of these women. Every detail is true. We haven't made anything up – we didn't need to. None of them is based on any one participant or Beyond Chocolater, so any details you might recognise are purely coincidental. All our characters are a melting pot, a blend of our own experience and that of all the women we have ever worked with.

We have grown very fond of these women over the months it has taken to write this book, and we hope you will like them too. They are your companions on this journey. We trust that they will inspire, guide and reassure you. The more we realise that we are not alone, that there are very few women out there who are effortlessly slim, who are normal around food and who eat, enjoy and move on, the easier it will be to stop beating ourselves up and begin to make real, lasting changes.

READY, STEADY, GO!

We have divided this book into three sections: 'Get Ready', 'Steady' and 'Go!'. As the title suggests, in 'Get Ready', we'll be doing some prep work and laying down a common framework from which to start. In 'Steady', we'll be looking at the many facets of overeating, making sure we cover all the bases before you are ready to go. And finally, in 'Go!' we'll be giving you the tools you need to go Beyond Temptation.

In each chapter, you will find a call to action, giving you practical suggestions to experiment with. We've also provided an 'Action Checklist' at the end of each chapter, each list building on the previous one. Keep coming back to them; they contain all the steps you need to take to stop overeating.

And remember Alice, Becky, Christine, Debbie, Emily, Fatima, Grace, Heather, Isabelle, Jane, Kate, Leila, Natasha, Olivia and Pam will be showing you how it's done. They are here to show you how it is possible to transform your relationship with food and feel good about the way you eat. None of these women is perfect, none of them ends up normal (whatever that means) or sorted, yet they all make profound changes in the way they eat. They are with you, every step of the way. Follow their lead and you can't go wrong.

Get Ready

Welcome to the beginning of the end. Before we even start thinking about stopping overeating there's some groundwork to be done. We need to get ready. We're going to explore overeating, understand it, unpick it, so that we are really clear about what it *is* and why we do it.

Since you are reading this book, it's likely that you have been overeating for some time – that overeating is a major part of your life. Expecting to stop, just like that, is unrealistic and sets you up for failure.

Let's say you've been taking the bus to work for years, and one day you decide you'd like to cycle instead, you're unlikely to get there in one piece if you don't do some prep work beforehand. You'd do some research, check out different models, map out your route, maybe go on a road-safety course or read a book about it, decide what clothes are most appropriate and figure out how long it will take. All of this before you've even hopped on to a bike. All major changes require some kind of preparation and that's what this section is about. The information you gather in the course of the next three chapters will prepare you to take the next step.

In Chapter 2 ('What is Overeating?'), we'll be asking you to think about what the term overeating means to you. From nibbling to bingeing, we all have our pet names for a behaviour which *we* call overeating. What do *you* call

➜

it? In Chapter 3 ('Why Do We Do It?'), we'll be helping you work out why you overeat, so that you know exactly what your triggers are. Once you *know* why you overeat – not just why you think you do it – you are one step closer to working out how to stop. And, in Chapter 4 ('Lighten the Load'), we will be inviting you to look at how the shame and the secrecy that go hand and hand with overeating weigh you down and keep you stuck, and we'll show you how to lighten the load, so you are free to move forward.

IMPORTANT INFORMATION

It is essential that you *allow* yourself to overeat while you work through this process. Use each time you overeat as an opportunity to learn something of value, which will ultimately help you stop. If you stop overeating too soon, you'll be missing out on vital information.

It is only when you are willing to acknowledge your overeating, to stop fighting it, to make friends with it, to learn from it, that you are free to discover how to stop.

So, let's **GET READY!**

CHAPTER TWO

What is Overeating?

THERE ARE COUNTLESS WAYS of overeating and we all have different names for it. In this chapter, we'll be looking at how we trivialise our overeating with euphemisms, medicalise it with labels or justify and excuse it with metaphors. It's time to strip away the smoke screens and call overeating what it is. Recognising what we do and naming it is the first step.

EVERYONE DOES IT

Who hasn't had another slice of cake just because it's so delicious, a bar of chocolate to cheer themselves up, another helping of mashed potato, just because they fancy it? If you're reading this, the likelihood is that you are not one of the lucky few who overeat occasionally, enjoy it and move on.

For most of us overeating is a very different experience. It's what we do all the time, day in day out. We may enjoy it in the moment and instead of moving on, it sometimes feels like we're going round in circles. We feel guilty, ashamed or disgusted. If only we could stop, we know we'd be happier, healthier, more in control and possibly slimmer. But somehow, despite our best intentions, we just *can't.*

SO MANY WOMEN ... SO MANY WAYS OF OVEREATING ...

Overeating is an all-encompassing term which describes a myriad different experiences.

Alice walked out of the nutritionist's office and went straight to the supermarket to stock up on a giant jar of Nutella, brie, salami, dried mango strips, Kinder eggs, strawberry shoelaces, bread, butter and full-fat Coke. At home, she unpacked the goodies on the table and then **binged** her way through the pile.

Becky constantly **overdoes it** at meals. All the time, every day. She starts off with what she tells herself is a reasonable portion, but then she just can't stop. One helping leads to another and then another. She eats and eats until there's literally nothing left. Nothing on her plate. Nothing in the bowl and nothing in the pan.

Christine eats in secret. She walks around with pockets full of jelly beans, Smarties or M&Ms; anything small, that can be easily concealed in the palm of her hand. She eats them all day long, popping one in her mouth when no one is looking.

Debbie regularly throws a coat on, over her pyjamas and goes out to the petrol station late at night to buy the crisps and chocolates she is **craving**.

Emily stuffs herself with packs of cheese and salami in the car on the way home from the supermarket, cramming in the slices and stopping off before she gets back to throw away the evidence in the same bin every time.

Fatima waits until everyone has gone to bed and then she **raids the fridge, pigging out** on leftovers, eating quickly with her fingers.

Grace stayed at home on Saturday night and drowned her sorrows in a humongous bowl of caramel popcorn and gallons of chocolate milk: the best food for **comfort eating**.

Heather went out of her way to pick up an extra-large Big Mac menu at the Drive-Thru, her **emotional eating** pitstop.

Isabelle is babysitting for the next-door neighbours. She is standing in front of their snack cupboard, agonising. Should she break the seal on a new pack of Garibaldis (she loves Garibaldis), and risk them knowing she's eaten their food or should she **sneak** the slightly stale digestives which aren't half as appealing? After weighing up the pros and cons she opts for the digestives. She reckons they won't notice – and they're easier to throw up.

Jane treats herself with food every time she has a moment away from the children and is always **picking** at bits of congealed fish fingers and soggy Marmite soldiers from their plates while she clears up after tea.

Kate thinks she's **addicted** to carbs. She has been laying off them for weeks. Resisting with iron will. But something in her snapped on Sunday and she **gave in** to roast potatoes, Yorkshire pudding and treacle tart at the pub and then carried on at home. To her horror, she ate every single one of the muffins she'd baked for her nephew's birthday party.

Leila works from home, **grazing** all day with repeated visits to the kitchen for a bit of this and bit of that: carrot sticks, a cup of tea and an oatcake, a handful of nuts, a low-fat yoghurt, a Diet Coke, an apple, a bowl of Special K, a couple of Ryvitas with Marmite and low-fat spread . . . more Diet Coke, more carrots . . . On and on, **eating all day**.

Natasha has finished a packet of Doritos only ten minutes into her favourite TV show. After a brief debate with herself, she dashes to the kitchen for another pack as soon as the adverts come on. There are another two packs in the cupboard, waiting. She knows she's a **compulsive eater** and doesn't know what to do about it.

Olivia ate four portions of cake at her sister's wedding. Everyone was **indulging** and having fun and nobody noticed her **stuffing herself**.

Pam eats too much at lunch in the canteen. She has the pudding every day, hungry or not – it's included in the meal and everyone else has one.

OVEREATING IS OVEREATING

Whether you're grazing on carrot sticks and rice cakes all day in an effort to stay away from the chocolate, or you overdo it at meals with yet another helping of pasta or methodically binge your way through your kitchen: it's overeating.

We will be using the term **overeating** throughout this book because it's factual. It simply describes a behaviour. In the dictionary, overeating is defined as: 'to eat to excess, especially when habitual. To eat more food than our body needs.' There's no moral judgment attached to it; it's a neutral description.

When we give the overeating we do inconsequential names like grazing and treating ourselves we trivialise it, or brush it under the carpet. We can pretend that everything is fine really. Some of us label it as bingeing or compulsive eating and surrender our power to a disorder over which we have no control. When we call it pigging out or stuffing ourselves we are judgmental, and that's how we paralyse ourselves in a sticky web of guilt and shame.

TAKE ACTION

Taking action is how we make changes. Whether you are changing a behaviour or changing the way you think, you're taking action. Start here:

Action 1

Your first action is to make it official and name it.

What names do you give your overeating? Look at

→

the list below of terms most commonly used to describe overeating and for each one ask yourself:

- Do I use this term to describe how I overeat?

- What does it tell me about how I think of my overeating?

- Do I consider this overeating?

You may also have your own, very personal names for overeating. Make sure you add these to the list.

Compulsive eating	Giving in
Emotional eating	Eating all the time
Grazing	Eating all day
Picking	Pigging out
Overdoing it	Stuffing myself
Overindulging	Treating myself
Addicted to . . .	Eating too much
Indulging	Sneaking food
Constant nibbling	Eating in secret
Cravings	

....

....

....

→

Action 2

Start to notice the different ways in which you overeat. Be curious. When you find yourself overeating – by any name – call it just that. Stick to the facts.

Imagine you are creating a documentary about yourself. Become the David Attenborough of overeating. Find a place to record your field notes. There are endless possibilities. You can do it in a notebook, on random pieces of paper that you store in one place, on your computer or online. You can write a stream of consciousness, whatever is going through your mind, without thinking about it, or have a structure. You can keep a log, you can write regularly – every day or every week – or just whenever you feel like it. Here are some suggestions.

- Journal
- Spreadsheets
- Spider diagrams
- Blog
- Posting on a forum
- Voice recording
- Video diary

The purpose of this action is *not* to shame you into stopping. The goal is for you to become aware of what you do.

→

YOUR **ACTION** CHECKLIST

☐ **Make it official:** call it overeating

☐ **Observe yourself with curiosity:** overeat with awareness

•

CHAPTER THREE

Why Do We Do It?

IN THIS CHAPTER, WE'LL BE identifying all the reasons *why* we overeat. In order to stop overeating, we need to know exactly what purpose it serves in the first place. We can't change that which we don't understand.

DEBUNKING THE MYTH

We know it's bad for us. It's bad for our health, it limits our social life, it impacts on our relationships, it gets in the way of everything. It sucks up our energy, our money, our time and, ultimately, our happiness. We become secretive, sometimes we lie, to ourselves and to others. We feel guilty, ashamed, out of control and we end up hating ourselves and hating our bodies.

So why do we do it?

MYTH: I overeat because I'm lazy and greedy. I have no will-power. I am weak and pathetic and I have no self-control. All I need to do is get a grip, resist temptation, make healthy choices and eat less. I only have myself to blame. I know what to do – I just have to bite the bullet and do it. If I really wanted to, I would.

REALITY: You are no more weak, lazy or out of control than anyone else. Whether it shows or not, everyone has a coping mechanism of some kind. Yours happens to be overeating.

Food is a coping mechanism

It supports, it comforts, it soothes, it delights, it distracts, it numbs, it makes us socially acceptable. We overeat as a way of avoiding everything that's uncomfortable and challenging: our feelings, our thoughts, our lives. Overeating is a very effective way of coping with all the challenges of life. It works.

Food is everywhere

Food is legal, cheap and accessible. We can buy or make it whenever we want and it doesn't have to cost a fortune. We don't have to hide in an alleyway and risk arrest for a chocolate muffin. It's a central part of our everyday lives. We eat for fuel, but we also eat to socialise and to celebrate.

Overeating is a reaction to dieting and deprivation

We know only too well about portion control, healthy eating and exercise. Most of us have been on so many diets we could write books about it, but all that doesn't work for long. In fact, overeating is often a natural consequence of the deprivation of dieting. Whether you're dieting or not, if you consistently deny your hunger, skip meals, go hours without eating, deprive yourself of the foods you really want, then you are far more likely to overeat. Once you start eating, you can't stop. Eating when you're hungry, responding to your body's hunger cues, is just one of the ways to stop overeating.

It's the natural choice for 'Superwoman'

Food is the easiest way of getting some instant gratification, of doing something nice for ourselves. Eating is the best way to take a break or have a rest without actually stopping. It's a little window of pleasure in days that are otherwise filled with putting other people's needs before our own. Women tend to look after everyone else and put themselves at the bottom of the pile. We are dedicated to our jobs, to our children, we're supportive friends, sisters, daughters, partners, so much so, that there is often very little left for us. That chocolate muffin is often the only way we know to look after ourselves without putting anyone out, letting anyone down, going out on a limb or saying no.

SO MANY WOMEN ... SO MANY REASONS ...

We overeat for all sorts of reasons. They can be the same every time or change from day to day, or even hour to hour. Let's take a look at some of those reasons.

Alice overeats because it feels as though if she didn't eat she'd explode.

Becky overeats because it tastes soooo good and she doesn't know how to say no to herself.

Christine overeats because she needs something in her mouth all the time; it's reassuring and keeps her calm.

Debbie overeats because she can't hold out any longer and the crisps and chocolates she's trying so desperately to avoid and telling herself she shouldn't have beckon her irresistibly. One bite, one square is not enough. By the time she gives in to the craving, she just can't stop.

Emily overeats because people often comment about her weight and she's embarrassed to eat in front of others. Once she's on her own in the car, it's as if the floodgates open and she just can't stop herself.

Fatima overeats every night because she's ravenous from sticking to the tiny portions dictated by the diet plan. By the time she gets to the fridge, no amount of food seems to satisfy her hunger.

Grace overeats because she's sad or lonely, anxious or depressed and she just doesn't know how to make herself feel better in any other way. While she is eating she can forget everything. She can focus on the hit of sugar, the crunch of the crisps, the creaminess of the chocolate. Even when what she's eating stops tasting good, the action of chewing and swallowing, chewing and swallowing, mouthful after mouthful creates a temporary void – a bit like white noise – where for a moment, just for a moment, nothing else matters.

Heather overeats because she thinks another hamburger won't make any difference anyway. She tells herself she doesn't *deserve* to be thin. And while she's eating she has a fleeting moment of respite from hating herself.

Isabelle overeats because she's supposed to be on a diet, but she can't resist. Once she starts, she can't stop: who knows when she'll next get the chance to eat all those lovely treats?

Jane overeats because she tells herself she deserves it. Looking after the children on her own all day is such hard work. A little bit of something nice feels like a just reward.

Kate overeats because she thinks she's addicted. She tells herself that going anywhere near wheat or sugar means she won't be able to stop – that it does something to her body and that she'll just want more and more. So she gives them up . . . and eventually, hours, days weeks or even months later, ends up giving in.

Leila overeats to avoid having to do all those things on her endless 'to-do' list which she doesn't really fancy doing: finishing that report, writing that email, phoning that client.

Natasha overeats just because. It's what she does when she watches TV or reads a book, when she travels, when she's in good company or alone.

Olivia overeats because she doesn't know what else to do with herself, especially when she's with other people. Eating gives her something to do, so she doesn't have to stare into space with no one to talk to.

Pam overeats because it would be terribly rude and wasteful not to. How can she say no and waste good food when someone's gone to so much trouble for her?

IDENTIFYING WHY WE OVEREAT

Sometimes we know exactly why we are overeating. We can pinpoint a specific trigger. At other times, it's more subtle, and it's more difficult to make sense of it. It feels like we are overeating simply because we like the food and it tastes nice or because we fancy a bit of something sweet or savoury. Deep down though, we know there's more to it, but we can't put our finger on the reason.

Sometimes it feels like we are on automatic pilot. No rhyme or reason. It's just what we do. We don't know why we ended up with our hand in the biscuit tin, again, we just did. Sometimes if feels like food is the only thing that helps us cope with life in general.

Whatever the reason, although overeating helps us feel better in the moment, we usually feel guilty or ashamed straight afterwards. We feel bad because we tell ourselves that we are weak, out of control, fat, lazy, greedy, stupid, selfish – fill in the blank. We subscribe to the myth. We are so busy beating ourselves up for overeating that we have no time or energy to look at what really is causing the distress. And sometimes that's the very reason we overeat.

OVEREATING HAS A POSITIVE FUNCTION

You may think that overeating is self-sabotage or a bad or unhelpful thing you do. And yet, while that may be true, overeating also has a positive function. It is a coping mechanism and, as such, it helps in the moment: it soothes away uncomfortable feelings, provides comfort in times of distress and distracts us from having to face the unfaceable. It helps us cope with the ups and downs of life and, in the short term, that's a good thing.

Beginning to see our overeating as a coping mechanism that we have developed for good reasons is vital. For some of us, this coping mechanism is old. It goes back many years and the overeating becomes habitual. As adults we don't even need a specific trigger to set us off. The unease, the tension, the fear, the self-hatred we live with are all so ingrained and unconscious that eating is the way we respond to life.

Whatever the reason, the key is to acknowledge, with compassion and kindness, that we are looking after ourselves the best way we know how. When we stop criticising and condemning ourselves – when we stop fighting – we have the space to take a step back and start to see what's really going on.

Whatever lies behind your overeating is the key to stopping. And that's exciting because once you find out, you have the power to stop for good.

TAKE ACTION

Find out as much as you can about *why* you overeat. Your aim is to gather as much information as possible.

Notice if there are any specific overeating triggers: situations, people, places. And after you overeat, look back and take a moment to ask yourself these questions:

- What function was the food serving in that moment?

- What was it helping to manage or avoid?

Even when you have no idea of the reason or the function, or there appears not to be one, make a note of *that*. A pattern will emerge. Habitual behaviours tell us something about ourselves. If you just can't work out why you're eating, this in itself is a clue.

Now is not the time to *stop* overeating. If you don't let yourself do it, you won't discover what lies behind it. Overeat with awareness.

YOUR **ACTION** CHECKLIST

☐ **Make it official:** call it overeating

☐ **Observe yourself with curiosity:** overeat with awareness

☐ **Identify your triggers:** find out why you overeat

•

CHAPTER FOUR

Lighten the Load

DO YOU HAVE ANY IDEA just how many women overeat? Not just a little bit every now and then, but the kind of overeating that we feel ashamed of, that we hide from friends, colleagues and family. The kind of overeating that we would be mortified if anyone found out about. The overeating that we think is disgusting, out of control, crazy . . .

So many of us do it. The most damaging thing about it is the guilt and the shame that we carry around with us like a heavy rucksack on our backs. What makes overeating so painful, so agonising, is the way we torture ourselves about it and keep it secret. And it's the secrecy that perpetuates the shame and the pain.

Have you ever talked about your overeating, or is it a secret? Have you ever talked about your overeating, in detail, with your mates, your mum, your sister or your partner? Do you mention it at all? Maybe you make light of it, pass it off as inconsequential, allude to it without going into detail about how you really feel, or maybe you avoid talking about it altogether. Do you talk about what it's really like to be out of control, desperate to feel normal? Mostly, we stay silent, we hide, we collude with each other and keep the secret. The idea of talking honestly and openly about our overeating and how we feel about it is horrifying.

SO MANY WOMEN ... SO MANY SECRETS ...

Put two or more women in a room together and the conversation invariably turns to food, diets, weight loss, exercise, dress size. These topics seem to be at the centre of every conversation, and nobody ever talks about what it's *really* like. What's really going on. We stick to the safe, the superficial, the self-deprecating.

If only they knew what we were really thinking . . .

Alice

What she says: 'Power Plate is great. I kind of stopped for a while, but look at these thighs! I'm starting again on Monday.'

What she's thinking: You don't understand. As soon as I stop exercising, I turn to flab and I have to be really careful with what I eat. I can eat a bit more with Power Plate because it burns loads of calories . . . but it's so tiring.

Becky

What she says: 'Do you want this box of Celebrations? I've got to get rid of them. I can't have them in the house or I'll eat them all!'

What she's thinking: I've been pretending to myself that I'm stocking up on boxes of chocolates in preparation for Christmas – they are only ten pounds for two at Sainsbury's at the moment. But it's not true. I sit there and eat a whole box every night in front of the telly.

Christine

What she says: (*Apologetically, as she tucks into a waffles and ice cream*) 'Yeah, I know, I'm really lucky. I inherited my mum's metabolism. I burn everything I eat.'

What she's thinking: If only you knew. All I eat is sweets. I haven't had a proper meal in ages.

Debbie

What she says: (About a helping of mashed potato) 'Oh no, thanks. I'm being good.'

What she's thinking: Oh no, I can't. Do you have any idea what I did last night? I threw the chocolate cake in the bin, but I went back, picked it out and had it anyway. Oh God! Why am I so out of control?

Emily

What she says: 'I don't understand how I managed to put on so much weight in the last year. It's not as if I eat a lot or anything. I may have the odd pie now and again but really . . . '

What she's thinking: But really . . . I have pies all the time. I can't stop eating. I can't.

Fatima

What she says: (*Tugging at her waist*) 'Urggh! I hate this bit here, it's disgusting! I've got to stick to that diet.'

What she's thinking: Sometimes I dream I'm sawing pieces of myself off. Isn't that really awful? I just can't stick to that sodding diet. I just can't stop the midnight binges.

Grace

What she says: 'Go ahead without me, I've got to finish this. I'll grab a sandwich later.'

What she's thinking: I can't go out to lunch with you. I've been eating all weekend. I didn't go out of the house except to stock up. I'm so lonely.

Heather

What she says: 'Wow! You look great! Have you lost weight?'

What she's thinking: You lucky cow, I'm just getting fatter and fatter. My clothes are really tight and I feel sick and bloated all the time. I can't stop eating . . .

Isabelle

What she says: 'My God, did you see Victoria Beckham on telly last night? She looks like a stick insect, she's so thin. Ugh!'

What she's thinking: I'd give my back teeth to look like that. I wish I had the willpower to starve like she does.

Jane

What she says: (*Reaching for another biscuit*) 'Look at me, aren't I being naughty, oh dear.'

What she's thinking: I can't believe I did this, but last night I ate all the sweets out of my son's birthday party bags. Now I'm going to have to buy more. How did it get to this?

Kate

What she says: 'No thanks. It looks lovely, but I'm trying to be more healthy.'

What she's thinking: You wouldn't believe how many wine gums I shovelled down my throat yesterday. My God! The e-numbers, the sugar, the gelatine . . . why do I eat that kind of thing?

Leila

What she says: 'Slimming World is brilliant; you can eat as much as you like!'

What she's thinking: I feel so bad. Yesterday I ate a whole family pack of Kettle Chips, some crackers and hummus and a tub of olives before dinner. By the time Mark got home I wasn't hungry, but he hates eating on his own, so I sat down with him and ate a whole plate of roast chicken, potatoes and veg and even shared a chocolate pudding with him afterwards. I feel so guilty.

Natasha

What she says: 'Oh, go on then – it does look lovely.'

What she's thinking: I can't believe I'm still eating. We went out for Chinese last night and I really pigged out. I wasn't particularly hungry, but everyone was enjoying it and tucking in and the conversation was great. I just couldn't stop. I felt so sick afterwards and I still had an ice cream at the cinema. I knew I shouldn't have had it; I was way past stuffed.

Olivia

What she says: 'Mmmmm . . . '

What she's thinking: I know you all think I'm weird. You don't know what it's like to be fat. Sometimes I wish I was dead.

Pam

What she says: 'I've decided to have another go at Weight Watchers. The new plan sounds really good and my friend has lost a stone already.'

What she's thinking: I'm desperate. I know Weight Watchers doesn't work – I've been a member for six years. Bingeing and starving myself to lose and put on the same two stone. But I just don't know what else to do.

OUTING IT

The more we are willing to talk about what it's really like, to stop keeping it a secret and to normalise what is, in reality, such a widespread experience among women, the less ashamed and alone we feel. Shame and secrecy keep us locked into a vicious cycle of self-loathing and sabotage: the more we blame and criticise ourselves for overeating, the more we overeat to numb the pain. So when we stop feeling so bad about ourselves, it's no big surprise to discover that we are less inclined to overeat. When we are more honest with others we are also more honest with ourselves. Having integrity feels good. And when we feel good, we eat less.

You may be surprised by other people's reactions. Courage and honesty tend to elicit admiration and respect. When we feel admired and respected, we feel good. And, once again, when we feel good, we overeat less.

When we tell the truth, we give other people permission to do the same. We empower and inspire them. And that feels good too. And, yet again, when we feel good about ourselves we are less inclined to overeat . . .

It may seem strange to suggest that talking openly about the way we overeat can be an act of courage, integrity and empowerment. And yet overeating and being fat are this generation's biggest taboos. Just a couple of decades ago, few women would have felt comfortable talking openly about being in debt, being gay or being on antidepressants. It's thanks to those who had the courage to speak up that it's so much easier to talk about these things today.

It's time to break the overeating taboo, and the only way to do that is to break the silence and start talking. When we can openly talk about the challenges of our relationship with food and our bodies, without putting ourselves down or pretending it's all fine, the world will be a better place for it.

TAKE ACTION

Are you weighed down by shame, guilt, self-criticism and disgust? Do you imagine that there's no one who's as messed up with food as you are, that no one stoops as low as you do, that some of the things you've done are so disgusting, so out of control, so awful that no one would understand? Think again.

Every time you overeat and beat yourself up and feel guilty or ashamed about it, it's like adding another rock to the heavy sack you carry around on your back. Find a place to dump the shame – to get rid of it. Here are a few ideas on how you can do this:

- Log on to the Beyond Chocolate Forum. There are hundreds of women there who all know what it's like because they do it too. Women who come on our workshops and members of the online community invariably tell us how liberating it is to talk openly with other women who won't judge them about their relationship with food and their bodies, and what the struggle is really like. Hearing (and reading) things that they have never dared say out loud is reassuring and comforting beyond words. Log on and post about your overeating. Share it and then leave it behind.

→

- Is there anyone you trust who you can talk to? A friend, a family member, a colleague? Someone who you have an inkling will understand and not judge you? If so, tell them about your relationship with food. Tell them what you are doing about it too. You may be surprised at the response.

- For the brave or militant among you, visit the Beyond Chocolate Facebook page and post your overeating stories. It's a place to dump the shame and leave it behind. There are already many stories there, including ours. Add yours and get rid of the shame. You don't need it any more. It doesn't serve you in any way. Lighten the load. You'll find it easier to move forward.

And if the whole idea of talking about it – outing yourself – is too big a step, start here: stop eating in secret. Stop hiding your overeating. Stop hiding it from *yourself*.

YOUR **ACTION** CHECKLIST

☐ **Make it official:** call it overeating

☐ **Observe yourself with curiosity:** overeat with awareness

☐ **Identify your triggers:** find out why you overeat

☐ **Lighten the load:** talk about what it's really like

Steady

In the previous chapters, we laid down the foundations for the work we'll be doing in this section. We have shed light on overeating, we've normalised it. We've given it a name. We've owned it. We have accepted and acknowledged that it serves a purpose right now and that it's nothing to be ashamed of. Now we're standing on solid ground. We are ready to take the next step. There's more work to be done before we are ready to GO. This section of the book is all about understanding the mechanics of overeating, and we do this by tuning in.

TUNING IN: A SIMPLE AND EFFECTIVE TOOL

We live in a society that makes it so easy to tune out. Whether we are busy all the time or empty and alone, tuning out is what we know best. We tune out by spending hours online or watching telly, we tune out with a glass of wine (or two or three), we tune out with exercise, with shopping and, of course, we tune out with food. Now it's time to tune *in*.

Tuning in is a straightforward and effective information-gathering tool which will give you an instant reading of where you're at – from an intellectual, emotional and physical perspective – in any given moment. It's a simple three-step process which takes less than a minute.

→

Whatever the overeating trigger, we respond with our thoughts, our feelings and our bodies. Tuning in is the best way to understand how we do this. And, as we saw in the previous section, awareness is crucial; if we don't know what we are doing, we can't change anything. Tuning in makes it possible to become aware of our thought process, to identify how we are feeling and to recognise how we embody the things we are experiencing.

And the good news is that once we have this information, we can make a conscious choice to change any one of these responses and, therefore, the whole dynamic, so that our triggers don't automatically lead to overeating.

Tuning in is the cornerstone of the Beyond Temptation approach.

✦

In Chapter 5 ('Resistance is Futile'), we'll be looking at why so often, it's the very foods we tell ourselves we should avoid that we end up overeating. Chapter 6 ('The Overeating Gremlin') reveals how the way we think and the things we tell ourselves can lead us to the biscuit tin. In Chapter 7 ('The Emotional Eater'), we'll explore how our feelings are intricately linked with the way we eat. And in Chapter 8 ('The Overeating Body') we'll delve into the physical, to discover how our bodies talk and

→

what this has to teach us about our overeating. We'll then be inviting you to play, yes play, with the idea of stopping overeating in Chapter 9 ('The Pause'). Consider this a sort of dress rehearsal. By the end of this section, you will have all the information, awareness and experience you need to use the tools that you'll find in the last section of the book.

So, **STEADY** —
we're not quite ready
to go just yet.

•

CHAPTER FIVE

Resistance is Futile

DEPRIVATION AND DIETING, trying to be good, being careful, counting calories or points or 'syns', watching what we eat, all lead to overeating. It doesn't matter why we deprive ourselves or what we deprive ourselves of; whether we avoid cake because we think it's fattening or burgers because we think they are unhealthy, the very fact of limiting ourselves and trying to avoid or cut down on the foods we like and want to eat, practically guarantees that we will crave them and then overeat them at some point.

And whether we actually deprive ourselves of our forbidden foods or just tell ourselves constantly that we shouldn't be eating this or that and then end up eating it anyway – it all adds up to the same thing. The diet and deprivation mentality persists, even when we have stopped dieting and officially depriving ourselves. If we feel in any way that we shouldn't be eating something, we will feel deprived. And when we feel deprived, we overeat.

In this chapter, you'll begin to see how having a list of forbidden (bad, naughty, fattening) foods which you try to avoid or eat only in moderation, impacts your overeating. Have you ever found yourself trying hard to resist that bar of chocolate or slice of cake, using every ounce of willpower you have only to give in minutes, hours or even days later? And then, once you've surrendered to temptation, it feels like one just isn't enough . . . or two, or three. Before you know it, you're overeating and promising to start again and be good tomorrow. The moment the chocolate passes your lips it's as if the floodgates open and your desire can feel insatiable.

SO MANY WOMEN ... SO MANY FORBIDDEN FOODS ...

Alice feels very strongly about the environment. She wants to do her bit to reduce the carbon footprint and avoids produce that isn't grown locally. She loves mangoes, pineapples and coconuts which, sadly, don't grow anywhere in the UK. Last week, she couldn't face another apple, pear or plum and, as if in a trance at the supermarket, she found herself in front of the exotic fruits, guiltily piling all her favourites into her basket. At home she ate all of them in one go, quickly, standing up at the kitchen counter, desperate to get rid of them. She felt so guilty and ashamed; how could she be so weak and irresponsible?

Becky keeps on promising herself she's going to start being good tomorrow. It's her mantra. Meanwhile, she eats chocolate, cakes, biscuits, crisps – all her favourite naughty foods – in anticipation of the deprivation to come.

Christine doesn't officially eat sweets. She's a dentist so she should, and does, know better. Thing is, she just can't help herself. And the more she tries to avoid them, the more she eats them. She's had to cut down drastically on proper meals to maintain her weight. She's practically living off sweets.

Debbie won't go near cakes, biscuits or chocolate. She's sure she puts on weight just looking at them! She refuses politely when offered, steers clear of dangerous supermarket aisles and always goes for low-fat, low-calorie or diet options. Until she just can't resist any longer, then she finds herself late at night raiding the petrol station for Mars bars, Cadbury's mini rolls, Galaxy bars, Kit Kats, Hobnobs, chocolate milk and brownies. She sits in her kitchen in the dark eating, eating, eating until it's all gone and she's surrounded by wrappers and remorse.

Emily regularly devours packets of salami and cold frank-furters on her way home from the supermarket in the car. She's *supposed* to be vegetarian and most of the time it's ok; just sometimes though, she can't resist and ends up giving in and bingeing on anything meaty.

Fatima loves food, but her father is a doctor and he's put her on another diet. She sticks to the rules when he's around and is really good, then, as soon as he turns his back, she eats anything tasty she can get her hands on.

Grace gave up diets a while ago. Nothing made a difference anyway, so she figures she might as well eat. She knows she shouldn't, that she's just getting bigger and that she should eat less sugar and fat. But she can't seem to care enough, and the food tastes so good. She's horrified, but just can't seem to do anything differently.

Heather thinks that fast food is really unhealthy. She tells herself she can't have the double cheeseburger, fries and Coke she really fancies. Somehow though, she regularly ends up at the Drive-Thru on her way home from work, stuffing down one or even two meal deals, feeling crap and swearing she won't do it again.

Isabelle's mum thinks it's indulgent to spend a lot of money on food and always chooses the cheapest or best-value meals. Isabelle has to eat what her mother puts on the table, even if that's not what she really fancies. Then later, she finds herself rooting around the cupboards for something – anything – nice that will satisfy her.

Jane never buys crisps. If her children see her eating them, they'll want some and she wants to set a good example. The problem is, she loves them (especially Walkers cheese and onion) and often buys herself a multi-pack on her way home from dropping them off at school. It's her guilty secret.

Kate tries really hard to avoid refined carbs and sugar. She keeps on reading about how addictive they are and how it can help with weight loss to cut them out. She does really well for a few days and sometimes for weeks at a time and then she loses the plot. Last time she went back to her parents for a weekend, she ended up eating masses of her mum's scones with cream, ice cream, pasta bakes and toast with butter . . . she just couldn't stop.

Leila's husband is allergic to dairy products, so she has excluded them completely and adapted her cooking to manage without them. As soon as he's not there for dinner though, she seizes the opportunity to treat herself and has a dairy feast, polishing off bowls of creamy pasta, cheese and biscuits and ice cream. She just can't get enough and she has to finish it all because even the smell of it in the fridge nauseates him.

Natasha doesn't officially eat sweets and snacks. She never buys them as part of her regular weekly shop at the supermarket. But despite her best intentions, she finds herself browsing the confectionery aisles online and guiltily stores the deliveries under her bed.

Olivia knows she eats too much and is constantly battling with herself to reduce her intake. She starts out every morning with good intentions: to have a healthy breakfast, a light lunch and something low-calorie for dinner. But then there's always some crisis at the office or at home and she ends up overeating chocolates and crisps and anything that tastes good, vowing to start properly again tomorrow.

Pam believes that the best way for her to lose weight is to stick to an eating plan and eat sensibly, so that she knows exactly how many calories she is eating at each meal and she makes sure she gets a balanced diet. She does pretty well for a week or so, and once, she lasted three entire months. More often than not though, she gets so bored that she ends up gorging on Chinese takeaways, just to taste something nice.

WHAT YOU RESIST PERSISTS

There are many different reasons why the foods we deprive ourselves of end up on a forbidden-foods list. The number-one reason is usually that they are regarded as fattening. These are some of the other reasons we've heard over the years:

✦ It's too expensive and self-indulgent

✦ It's unethical

✦ It's unhealthy

✦ It's junk

✦ It's too childish

✦ No one else in my family eats it

✦ I've been told I have an intolerance

And so on . . .

Whatever the reason, the more we tell ourselves we can't or shouldn't or mustn't have something, the more likely it is that at some point we will give in to temptation and end up eating more of it than we want or need.

Identifying all the foods we don't allow ourselves to eat freely or without guilt gives us a starting point for normalising our relationship with them. In this context, normal means allowing ourselves to eat what we want without the emotional and mental turmoil that so often goes hand in hand with deciding what to eat. Being able to have a piece of cake, just because we fancy it, without feeling bad about it or telling ourselves we've failed or that we'll have to make up for it somehow (by being good tomorrow or exercising for an extra ten minutes).

A normal relationship with food means feeling absolutely fine deciding *not* to have something we fancy without feeling deprived. And that can only come from knowing that nothing is forbidden. From knowing that we are allowed to eat whatever we want because it is our choice. There are no rules.

Choice is an amazing thing because it frees us to say no. It may sound counterintuitive, but it works. If we tell ourselves not to have something, we can't stop wanting it, as we know only too well. When we give ourselves permission, no holds barred – suddenly the compulsion is gone.

As you've been reading this, you may already have been making a mental list of all your forbidden foods. Some of them are obvious, and you know exactly what they are. And, sometimes, the more you think about it, the more foods will make their way on to the list, foods that aren't so obvious, but that, for some reason you restrict (or try to restrict). The first step in normalising your relationship with all foods is to identify your forbidden ones and why you try so hard to resist them.

TAKE ACTION

Action 1

Make a list of all your forbidden foods. These are any foods that:

- you deprive yourself of
- you try to eat in moderation

→

- you think of as unhealthy or fattening and, therefore, avoid

- you eat in secret

- you can't control yourself around

- you never buy

- you feel bad about eating

- you wish you could only have one

- you won't rest until they're eaten, if you have some in the house

- you have as a treat

- you think you're addicted to

- you were not allowed to eat (or had restricted) as a child

- you don't buy because they're expensive or indulgent.

Action 2

When you find yourself overeating any of the foods on your list, ask yourself these questions:

- Why is this food forbidden?

- Why did I choose this particular food?

- What do I like about this particular food?

- Does this food satisfy me and how much of it does it take to do so?

→

No forbidden foods?

If you really, truly don't have any forbidden foods, this chapter is not for you. Instead, focus on what we've been doing up to now.

YOUR **ACTION** CHECKLIST

☐ **Make it official**: call it overeating

☐ **Observe yourself with curiosity**: overeat with awareness

☐ **Identify your triggers**: find out why you overeat

☐ **Lighten the load**: talk about what it's really like

☐ **Find out about your forbidden foods**: make a list

•

CHAPTER SIX

The Overeating Gremlin

I T MAY SOMETIMES FEEL AS though we suddenly find ourselves with our hand in the biscuit tin or staring at an empty plate, without having thought about it at all. In fact, there is always a thought process that leads us to overeating. However briefly or unconsciously, we do talk ourselves into it.

We all have an internal dialogue – a continuous conversation with ourselves about all sorts of things. Often, these are half-baked thoughts, so unconscious that we don't even recognise them as such. They are fast and fleeting, far faster than speech. And importantly, the things we say to ourselves dictate how we feel and what we do.

And the dialogue goes on during and after we've overeaten too. We cajole, threaten, bully, shame, scare or comfort ourselves to the metaphorical (or actual) biscuit tin. And then we beat ourselves up for going there. We often fall into a spiral of self-criticism and blame. We rebuke ourselves and resolve to try harder, resist, stop it once and for all or we are resigned and despondent, like there's no way out.

By taking the time to tune in and pay attention to these thought processes we can slow them down enough to become fully aware of what we're saying to ourselves. This chapter is about learning to recognise and explore our internal dialogues, so that later on we can change the way we talk to ourselves and not end up overeating.

WE'D LIKE YOU TO MEET THE OVEREATING GREMLIN

Our Overeating Gremlin is the personification of our thinking, our internal dialogues and the beliefs we have about ourselves and the way we eat. It is one of the things that keeps us stuck in a pattern of overeating then beating ourselves up for it.

Some of you may be nodding as you read this; you understand exactly what we mean when we talk about dialogues, beliefs and Gremlins. If, on the other hand, you're unsure (or you think it sounds a bit odd), look at the list below, as you may know it by a different name:

✦ Top dog

✦ The voices in your head

✦ The tape

✦ The script

✦ Introjects

✦ Internal dialogue

✦ Limiting beliefs

- ✦ The inner critic
- ✦ The wounded child
- ✦ The inner saboteur
- ✦ The critical parent
- ✦ Subconscious messages
- ✦ The superego

We have Richard David Carson and his excellent book *Taming your Gremlin: A surprisingly simple method for getting out of your own way* to thank for the term 'Gremlin'. Carson is certainly not the first person to have talked or written about this subject, but the term Gremlin – an invisible, mischievous troublemaker – works particularly well in this context. So that's why we have adopted it.

Where Gremlins come from

We have picked up, developed and internalised these ways of talking to ourselves and these beliefs about life, about ourselves about our eating, over a lifetime.

As children, we were told things or witnessed the attitudes and behaviours of our parents, our carers, our teachers, friends, family members and society in general which we took on without questioning. When we look more closely at the dialogues we have with our Gremlin, we can often pick up echoes of an overprotective mother, a dominating father or a spiteful schoolmate. At other times, it is possible to link them to protection mechanisms that we created for ourselves in childhood that have persisted well beyond their usefulness. We made sense of the senseless and the confusing by creating truths and beliefs about ourselves and the world which matched our reality.

When we are children, it is far too scary for us to consider that the adults who are taking care of us are wrong, so we make *ourselves* wrong. Let's imagine you're five years old. You had your lunch fifteen minutes ago and now you're playing in the garden. You feel hungry, so you run into the kitchen and ask for something to eat. Your mum looks at you scornfully and says, 'Don't be silly' (or maybe she says, 'Don't be ridiculous', or 'greedy' or she shouts at you or ignores you or smacks you . . .). 'You just had lunch, you can't be hungry. Go out and play.' Aged five, you cannot believe that she is wrong and you are right. Despite the hungry feeling in your belly. She *has* to be right since she's the adult, the one who knows things, the one with experience. So, unconsciously, you decide that *you* are wrong. Since she knows better, you must be 'silly' or 'ridiculous' or 'greedy'. You *must* be. It's not wise or safe or helpful to be right. Regardless of the fact that you really did feel hungry, you learn not to trust your own body, not to listen to your needs, and you become very good at being critical or dismissive of yourself. Even if you were the type of child who had a tantrum and responded angrily to not having your needs met, unconsciously it's likely that you took on the belief that you were naughty or bad for being angry and for not doing what you were told without a fuss. It's what we do when we are little. It's normal. In fact, it's essential. These strategies serve us well when we are young; when we depend on others for our safety and our lives.

And, many of us continue to re-enact the strategies we developed as children in adulthood, and they become unconscious habits; we play the same tapes, buy into the same beliefs, live by the same rules. We keep telling ourselves that we are silly, ridiculous or greedy. And those beliefs become our Gremlins.

Let's look at another example of how this works.

Jemima and the Jelly Tots

Jemima is three and a half. She whizzes around the playground, up and down the slide, laughing and having fun. As she dashes towards the see-saw, she trips over, goes flying and ends up in a heap on the ground. She has a big graze on her knee. As she looks at the beads of blood, she bursts into tears. Within seconds, her mum is by her side. She scoops Jemima up, shushing and cuddling her, and pulls out a little bag of Jelly Tots from her pocket.

'Oh, don't cry sweetheart, don't cry. Here, have a little sweetie. Now let's clean you up. Do you want another one? Don't cry darling, it's just a little ouchie, it's nothing. Do you want to hold the packet while Mummy gets the wipes out?'

Is it any wonder that today Jemima tells herself not to cry, that it's nothing, and automatically turns to food when she feels pain or discomfort of any kind, emotional or physical? Her impulse is to soothe it away with food. This is Jemima's Overeating Gremlin at work.

This is not a blame game. Jemima's mum was doing her best. Our parents, carers and the other influential people in our lives usually have good intentions and don't set out to mess up our relationship with food. But being given food as a salve, a reward or a distraction, over and over again, eventually turns eating into our coping strategy of choice, lasting far beyond our playground days.

You and your Gremlins

Your Gremlin is a *part* of you – not *all* of you. It is a part of your mind at work. By tuning in and identifying it, and by recognising how it operates, how it talks and what it says, you can start to consciously shift the automatic and unhelpful behaviours it usually leads to.

Often, our habits and ways of talking to ourselves become so ingrained that we don't see them for what they are. We allow them to define us and think that this is just who we are. In fact, these are learned behaviours and, as such, they can be changed.

If we want to stop overeating, as well as the self-disgust and shame that almost always accompany it, it's time to stop submitting to our Gremlin and blindly following orders. While we are unconsciously being dictated to we have no choice. When we tune in and become conscious of our Gremlin and how it operates, we are no longer in its grip. We can decide who is in charge and who makes the decisions. We are no longer powerless in the face of our overeating. We no longer have to repeat the same destructive behaviours over and over again. We can begin to make *choices*. And tuning in is the key.

SO MANY WOMEN ... SO MANY GREMLINS ...

There are as many types of Overeating Gremlins as there are women who overeat. Each has a different tone, employs different tactics, has different beliefs and subscribes to different codes of conduct. No two are the same.

We each have our very own personal Gremlin. Some of them talk *to* us or at us ('You shouldn't do this; you mustn't eat that'), while others sound like our own voice ('I'm so greedy; I've got to get a grip'). Whatever their character, whether they are weak and pitiful or strong and bullying and whether they talk in the first or second person ('I' or 'you'), what they all have in common is that they have the power and we do their bidding.

Perhaps the most helpful way to explain what an Overeating Gremlin is and does is to show you what it's like in action.

Alice's holier-than-thou goody-goody

Alice's goody-goody won't let up. She insists on Alice being responsible, thinking of the consequences of her actions, and berates her constantly for not sticking to her principles. What would people think if they knew just how out of control the oh-so-professional lawyer really is?

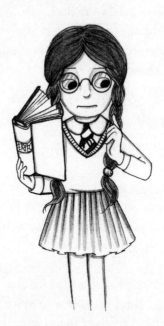

Overeating trigger

Alice has been to see the dietician and has lost two pounds. He's given her a new maintenance plan. On her way home she walks past a bakery . . .

Dialogue

Alice: Oh, that looks good.

Gremlin: No, you really shouldn't. But you have reached your target weight and, technically speaking, you don't have to start the new plan until Monday.

Alice: No, I really shouldn't.

Gremlin: It's only one doughnut. Just eat this and you'll start properly on Monday. Nobody needs to know.

Alice: No, but he said stay away from sugary things.

Gremlin: Well, from Monday you can do it really properly. No one will know. You had that fruit juice and that's sugary.

Alice: Oh, I don't know . . .

Gremlin: Look, you've messed it up already. Eat this, then start after the weekend. Weekends are always tricky; there's always something going on. What about the party tomorrow? You won't be able to stick to it then. Have the doughnut and you can make sure you stick to it really properly from next week.

Outcome

Alice eats three doughnuts.

Post-mortem

Gremlin: I don't see what the point is of going to the dietician and spending all that money, if you don't stick to it. It's not that hard, honestly.

◆ ◆ ◆

Becky's needy child

Becky's needy child clings to her desperately – whining and whimpering insistently for food. Becky soothes and quietens her with her favourite snacks, and then has to put up with the petulant, self-pitying remarks afterwards and always ends up feeling miserable and pathetic.

Overeating trigger

Becky is at a buffet. She's already piled her plate twice.

Dialogue

Gremlin: I want some more, I really want more.

Becky: Ooohhh.

Gremlin: No, but I really want it. I really, **really** want it . . . whimper . . .

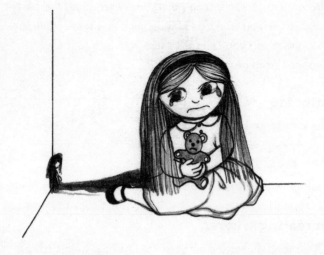

Outcome

Becky goes back for more.

Post-mortem

Gremlin: Whine, whine. It's not fair. I feel so sick. I want to go home.

✦ ✦ ✦

Christine's autopilot

Christine's autopilot sets the course and takes over. It directs her towards the food and Christine just eats. It doesn't say anything; there are no words. There's nothing to talk about. She's on autopilot.

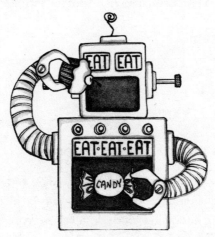

Overeating trigger

Another long day at the surgery. Two more patients to see before she goes home. Pocket full of jelly beans.

Dialogue

Gremlin: —

Christine: Chew, swallow

Gremlin: —

Christine: Chew, swallow

Gremlin: —

Christine: Chew, swallow

Gremlin: —

Christine: Chew, swallow

Gremlin: —

Outcome

Christine has a jelly bean and then another and then another.

Post-mortem

Gremlin: —

✦ ✦ ✦

Debbie's worn-out moaner

Debbie's moaner moans when she's on a diet, and moans when she's off a diet. Debbie's moaner goes on all the time, day in, day out about how hard and unfair everything and every-one is. When she's on a diet, she moans about how unfair it is that she's not allowed chocolate, and how boring that she has to eat the same, tasteless things every day. When she's off the diet, she moans about how fat she is and how ugly she looks.

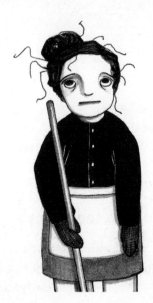

Overeating trigger

Filling up at the petrol station, waiting in the queue to pay.

Dialogue

Gremlin: I'm so fed up of Weight Watchers. I want some Galaxy. Oh, they're on offer. They would wait until I'm on a diet.

Debbie: Yeah. And the diet's not working anyway. I haven't lost anything this week.

Gremlin: Oh, it's so unfair. Why can't I be thin?

Debbie: I wonder what else I could have? Hmmm . . . cashew nuts?

Gremlin: They're fattening, anyway. Look at her, I bet she doesn't have to worry about what she eats. It's not fair, I want Galaxy.

Outcome

Debbie pays for her petrol and two bars of Galaxy.

Post-mortem

Gremlin: This is so hard! Oh God, I'm so fat. I'll never lose weight.

Emily's rebellious teenager

Emily battles unsuccessfully with her rebellious teenager. She comes at her from all directions, ranting and raving at the injustice of it all – sabotaging her every attempt at restraint and self-control. She dares her to eat more – just to show 'them' and gives her the finger when she looks in the mirror.

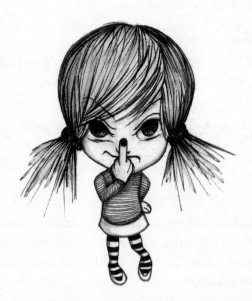

Overeating trigger

Standing in the cooked meats aisle at the supermarket.

Dialogue

Gremlin: Why should I care what anybody thinks. No one is telling me what I can or can't eat.

Emily: I'm vegetarian. I don't eat meat.

Gremlin: Yeah, so what? I want to.

Emily: But I'm supposed to be vegetarian.

Gremlin: Yeah, right. Who are you trying to kid? Just get it.

Emily: No, I really don't want to do this any more.

Gremlin: It's none of anybody's business if I want to have a bit of meat. Fuck them.

Outcome

Emily puts the pack of salami in her trolley.

Post-mortem

Gremlin: You're such a fraud.

Fatima's terrified twin

Fatima's terrified twin is constantly going into panic mode, dragging Fatima into her increasingly catastrophic scenarios about what will happen if she does eat . . . and what will happen if she doesn't. She's weak and pathetic and is always intent on showing Fatima just what a disaster her life is. Nothing and nobody can help. She drags Fatima towards food and then starts dreading the consequences.

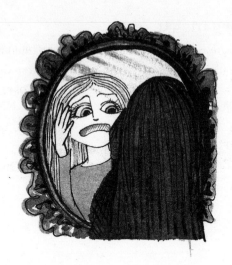

Overeating trigger

Standing in front of the open fridge after everyone has gone to bed, ravenous because she's eaten so little all day.

Dialogue

Gremlin: I can't do this. I'm starving. I'll never get to sleep. I haven't had anything proper to eat all day. I feel awful. I've got to have something.

Fatima: I can't. I've got to resist, otherwise I won't lose any weight and Daddy will know I've cheated.

Gremlin: I feel terrible, I can't cope. I have to eat. I think I'm going into famine mode. What if I faint? Oh God. What if they find me on the floor in front of the fridge?

Fatima: But if I start I won't be able to stop. Got to go back to bed.

Gremlin: No, I can't. I have to eat. Oh God, I hate this. I can't take it.

Outcome

Fatima eats some left-over cold roast chicken, then the potatoes, then a piece of cheese, then has some Coke, some pineapple chunks, more cheese, more Coke, more chicken . . . She just can't stop.

Post-mortem

Gremlin: He's going to find out; he'll be furious. Oh God, oh God, oh God.

✦ ✦ ✦

Grace's bullying dictator

Grace lives in a state of siege. Her bullying dictator comes down on her like a ton of bricks. His demands for food are loud, unrelenting and non-negotiable. He goes on and on until she gives in and then switches tack and shouts at her for being weak, pathetic and out of control.

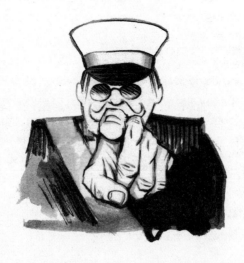

Overeating trigger

Being alone at home.

Dialogue

Gremlin: JUST HAVE IT!

Grace: Oh God.

Gremlin: I DON'T CARE. JUST HAVE IT.

Grace: Oh, I'm so tired of this. I want to be normal.

Gremlin: EAT AND GO TO BED. JUST FUCKING EAT IT.

Grace: Oh God.

Outcome

Grace eats.

Post-mortem

Gremlin: You're pathetic. You're fat. Sort yourself out.

Heather's vicious devil

Heather's devil criticises and puts her down all day long. He's cruel and spiteful and knows exactly what to say to make her feel awful. Sometimes he's loud and overbearing; other times he whispers maliciously in her ear. He goads her relentlessly into eating and then has a field day ripping her to shreds afterwards.

Overeating trigger

Being the fattest woman at the party.

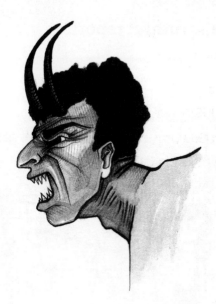

Dialogue

Gremlin: You're so weak. Look at you, you fat cow. You make me sick. You're pathetic. You always end up eating. No wonder you're the fattest one here. No one else does this. You are fat. FAT. FAT!

Heather: (Heather says nothing)

Outcome

Heather sits in the car eating.

Post-mortem

Gremlin: You're a failure. You're fat, you're disgusting, you make me sick. What is it with you? There's something really wrong with you. You deserve to be fat.

✦ ✦ ✦

Isabelle's truthful reporter

Isabelle's truthful reporter is matter of fact and sounds like she's just stating the obvious. She's detached and analytical and is forever coming up with universal truths about how and what Isabelle eats and what she looks like. She's relentless and won't engage in discussions. Her opinion is the last word. She knows best.

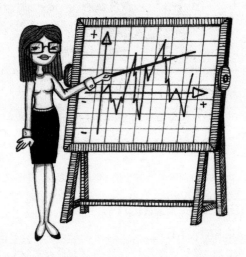

Overeating trigger

Yet another of her mum's horrible best-value meals.

Dialogue

Gremlin: Dinner was disgusting. You have to have something nice.

Isabelle: But they're really fattening.

Gremlin: No they're not. They're only twenty-five calories and you had 315 at dinner, so it's hardly going to make a difference. Look at you anyway, you're bum is so big you don't even fit into your fat jeans any more. Are you really telling me these three biscuits are going to tip the balance? Just eat them.

Isabelle: But I can't. I'll end up eating the whole pack. I know I will.

Gremlin: That's ok. You know what to do. It won't count at all.

Outcome

Isabelle eats the whole pack, then makes herself sick in the toilet.

Post-mortem

This is ridiculous. You're killing yourself. You've got to stop.

✦ ✦ ✦

Jane's damsel in distress

Jane's damsel is easily overwhelmed and is always telling her she can't cope, it's all too much, she doesn't know what to do and eating will make it all go away for a bit. Except that afterwards, Jane is left to deal with even more distress and despair.

Overeating trigger

At the supermarket on her own, for once.

Dialogue

Gremlin: I haven't stopped all day. I'm so tired. I deserve these, I really do. It's my only treat.

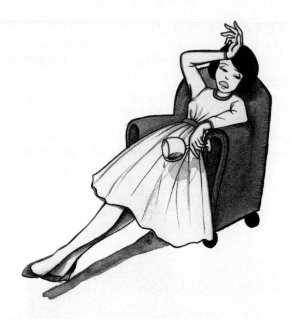

Jane: Maybe the small pack . . .

Gremlin: That won't be enough.

Outcome

Jane buys a multi-pack of Walkers cheese and onion crisps. She has two packs in the car on the way home, then another one while she's putting away the shopping and one more with a cup of tea.

Post-mortem

Gremlin: Oh no. What have I done? Four packets of crisps. Four.

✦ ✦ ✦

Kate's critical witch

Kate's critical witch finds fault with absolutely everything and has a running commentary on her shortcomings. Nothing she does is right. Stuffing food into her mouth is the only way to shut the hag up. But it's short-lived, and always followed by a disapproving deluge of criticisms and condemnations.

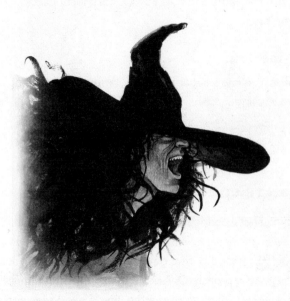

Overeating trigger

On a training course. After dinner in the hotel room.

Dialogue

Gremlin: Oh well done. Great self-control. Oh yeah, that's a really healthy diet. I mean, chocolate tart, what *were* you thinking? You didn't have to have it.

Kate: It was so good though.

Gremlin: Well, you might as well have these biscuits then. I mean, chocolate for chocolate.

Kate: I'll start again tomorrow and I'll ask them not to put any more of these in my room.

Outcome

Kate boils the kettle and eats all four hospitality packs of bourbon biscuits.

Post-mortem

Gremlin: You know sugar is poison. When are you going to stop eating it, once and for all?

Leila's relentless perfectionist

Leila's relentless perfectionist sets rigorously high standards which Leila invariably fails to live up to. She constantly urges her to try harder, do better, get it right, not let anyone down, to be beyond reproach. One slip is all it takes to set her off on a downward spiral of overeating. She's failed anyway, so today is spoiled. She promises herself she'll do it properly tomorrow . . .

Overeating trigger

An endless to-do list.

Dialogue

Gremlin: I've already messed it up for today, so there's no point trying to be good. I'll eat what I want today and

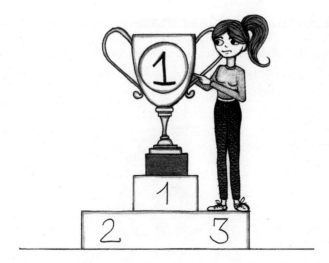

from tomorrow on I'll do it perfectly. I know I can do it. I'll definitely start tomorrow.

Leila: Ok then, just one more.

Gremlin: What's the point of just one? I've messed it all up for today, anyway.

Leila: Ok, just a few then.

Gremlin: Oh, I'll just take the whole packet, then I won't be tempted tomorrow.

Outcome

Leila takes the pack of cheese twists back to her desk.

Post-mortem

Gremlin: It's fine, tomorrow I'll make a fresh start and do it properly. I'm going to really do it perfectly. I really will.

◆ ◆ ◆

Natasha's reckless mate

Natasha's reckless mate has a carefree, 'what-the-heck' attitude to life and is forever urging her to loosen up, have fun, indulge and eat something nice.

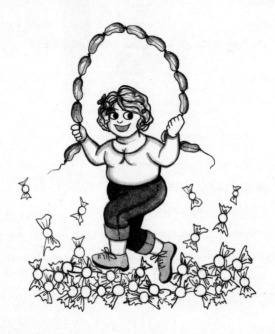

Overeating trigger

At a party.

Dialogue

Gremlin: Go on, let's have some fun! Lighten up! Whatever! Oh wow, look at all this stuff.

Natasha: I've just had dinner.

Gremlin: Oh, boring! Go on, it's nice. Who cares? So what? Look at those mini pavlovas, they're so dinky.

Natasha: I've put on loads of weight.

Gremlin: You know how to lose weight. Fuck it, go on. There's always Lighter Life.

Outcome

Natasha eats two mini pavlovas, a slice of chocolate torte, three mini cheese cakes and six chocolate truffles.

Post-mortem

Gremlin: Fuck it, life's too short.

✦ ✦ ✦

Olivia's black goo

Olivia's black goo is gelatinous. It hides in the recess of her brain and slithers around, hissing. It tries to swallow her up so she'll disappear. It tells her she doesn't belong, she shouldn't be here, nobody cares, she's not worth anything. Eating keeps her busy, so she doesn't have to listen to it.

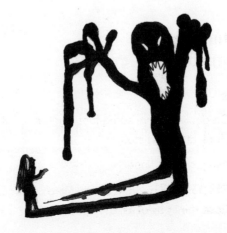

Overeating trigger

At her sister's wedding.

Dialogue

Gremlin: I want to disappear. I hate this. I don't belong.
I don't know what to say. Eating will give me something
to do.

Olivia: —

Gremlin: I can't bear it. I don't care, this is awful.

Olivia: —

Gremlin: Nothing can be worse than this. I shouldn't be here.

Outcome

Olivia eats four slices of wedding cake, sitting in a corner on
her own.

Post-mortem

Gremlin: I don't belong. Nobody loves me.

✦ ✦ ✦

Pam's reproachful granny

Pam's reproachful granny sits in the corner knitting and
mumbling reproaches under her breath. She never lets
Pam put herself first – it's rude and self-indulgent, she says.
She's a sour old bag who never lets Pam off the hook.

Overeating trigger

Sunday lunch at the in-laws.

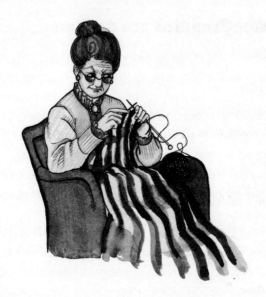

Dialogue

Gremlin: You can't refuse. That would be so rude.

Pam: Well, I don't really want it.

Gremlin: Yes, but it's just rude. She'll be so offended.

Pam: She *has* gone to a lot of trouble. But I feel so stuffed.

Gremlin: This isn't about you. Think of other people for a change.

Pam: Yes, yes I will have it.

Outcome

Pam accepts a large helping of her mother-in-law's treacle tart.

Post-mortem

Gremlin: You really did overdo it a bit at lunchtime. Time to show a little restraint.

Beware! Gremlins are devious

Your Gremlin wants to stay hidden; its job is to keep you stuck. *Your* job is to see it clearly, so that it sits squarely in front of you, face to face, eye to eye instead of hiding on your shoulder, crouching in your head, towering over you or standing in your way. Be vigilant! Your Gremlin is crafty and will find ways of sneaking up on you when you least expect it. It may start out with a perfectly friendly opening gambit, only to switch tactics once you're ensnared in the conversation, suddenly revealing its true nature.

For now, let it think it's in charge; continue to overeat – with awareness. Observe and be curious. Don't fight it or resist it. Instead, tune in, see it, catch it, notice it. Get to know it. Every time you overeat, you have an opportunity to tune in and really get to grips with your Gremlin.

How do I know if it's a Gremlin?

We have lots of thoughts and many internal dialogues or, indeed, monologues and they are not all Gremlins.

The way to tell if it's a Gremlin is to ask yourself if it's being helpful. Is what you do as a result of listening to it what you really want to be doing? If what you are 'talking yourself into' is something you are happy with, something you don't want to change, then it's not a Gremlin (even if it has echoes of a damsel in distress or a reproachful granny). Deciding to take a break and put your feet up because you are tired and fed up is not the same as deciding to delve into a pack of Hobnobs for the same reason. One is self-care, the other self-sabotage. (We've baptised the former the Fairy Godmother; she is the one who has your best interests at heart and knows what's really good for you.)

Your Gremlin is the one that keeps you stuck in old, destructive patterns, the one that won't be contradicted, the one that never gives up, thinks it knows best and wouldn't know the meaning of the word surrender if it hit it in the face.

But it's right!

So what if your Gremlin is telling you stuff that you agree with: you *should* be fitter; you *must* lose weight; you've *got* to stop overeating. You just *can't* afford to waste any more time; you *ought* to be able to sort this out; and you *absolutely have to* have a healthy diet. Surely everyone would agree that these are universal truths, wouldn't they? All of this might be true, everyone else might well agree and at the end of the day, true or not, it's not helpful to listen to these Gremlins. It never has been, you wouldn't be reading this book if it was.

The words 'ought to', 'must', 'should', 'can't', 'have to', 'got to', etc. are unhelpful because they are disempowering. They reduce us to naughty or pathetic little children who have to be told what to do.

If you truly believe that your Gremlin knows what it's talking about, then hang on to the belief and ditch the Gremlin. When you can say: I *want* to be fitter, I *want* to lose weight, I *want* to stop overeating, I *want* to do this now, I *want* to sort this out and I *want* a healthy diet – it becomes your decision. You don't have to be subjected to any type of bullying, hounding, lecturing and self-pitying to get what you *want*.

By tuning in and getting to know our Gremlins, seeing them for what they are, we take back the power – the power to make decisions. The power to stop overeating.

TAKE ACTION

The next time you overeat, tune in to your Gremlin. The best way to do this is by tuning in to your thinking, so that you begin to identify your Gremlin in action.

Often, we're eating before we know it, it happens so quickly. So aim to tune in as soon as you are aware that you are overeating or just after. In fact, it's helpful to tune in at any point.

Then, when you've done it once, plan to do it again. And again. Often. Practise – the more you do it, the better.

You may identify with more than one of the Gremlins described above. You may have both a needy child and a vicious devil and any other number of Gremlins which respond to different triggers and show up at different times and in different situations. For now, focus on one Gremlin at a time – the one that shouts the loudest or that demands your attention the most.

Tips for tuning in to your Gremlin

- Become aware of how your Gremlin talks to you and what it says. Is it:

  - Bullying
  - Angry
  - Critical
  - Nasty
  - Vicious

→

- Weak
- Needy
- Scared
- Seductive
- Patronising
- Matter of fact
- Silent

- Notice if your Gremlin has any favourite catchphrases.

- Notice how you react when your Gremlin starts playing up. How do you interact with it?
  - Do you answer back?
  - Do you collude with it?
  - Do you try to ignore it?
  - Do you just freeze and go on autopilot?
  - Do you follow orders and do what it says?
  - Do you eat to shut it up?
  - How long does it take for you to give in or give up and go along with it?

- In some cases, it may be a monologue, with the Gremlin doing its stuff and you mutely following orders.

- Although our ultimate objective is to put the Gremlin in its place and take charge, for now we are going to do quite the opposite. Know thine enemy, as they say. Your job is to tune in and welcome your Gremlin, tease it out, so that eventually you recognise it instantly and it does not catch you unawares. Your aim for now is to

→

be curious, to bring your Gremlin into your awareness, to become the watcher, to shine a light on your Gremlin in action.

• You may find it helpful to create a caricature of your Gremlin (as we have done in this chapter). Give it a name, draw it, write down a typical dialogue you have with it. Once it's really clear just what you're dealing with and you can start to say, 'Aha – Gotcha!' you'll be ready to move on to the next stage which is shutting it up and taking charge.

Note: if you notice that you are telling yourself that this is a pile of bollocks, that it will never work and that Gremlins don't exist – that will be your Gremlin talking.

YOUR **ACTION** CHECKLIST

☐ **Make it official:** call it overeating

☐ **Observe yourself with curiosity:** overeat with awareness

☐ **Identify your triggers:** find out why you overeat

☐ **Lighten the load:** talk about what it's really like

☐ **Find out about your forbidden foods:** make a list

☐ **Tune in to your Gremlin:** get to know it

•

CHAPTER SEVEN

The Emotional Eater

MANY OF US WOULD DESCRIBE ourselves as emotional eaters and since you're reading this, you may well be one of them. But what does that mean?

Everyone has feelings. We all have moments of feeling sad, angry, anxious, excited. And yet, for a variety of reasons, we can find it difficult to recognise and express our emotions. When *feeling* is not something we are comfortable with, we may turn to overeating as a way to drown our sadness, to silence our anger, to quell our excitement, to numb our fears. Finding a way to deal with our emotions in a way that feels ok and manageable is central to stopping overeating. The first step is to identify and name what we are feeling by tuning in, and that's what we'll be doing in this chapter. The point of naming your feelings is not to stop you overeating just yet; it is to become aware of how your feelings lead you to the biscuit tin.

ANGRY, SAD, AFRAID, HAPPY

There are a myriad ways to describe how we feel, just like there are many names for overeating. When we dramatise or play down our feelings, when we use euphemisms or metaphors to describe them, we can feel overwhelmed or brush them off. We find it very helpful to divide our feelings into four categories: anger, sadness, fear and happiness. Being factual, non-judgmental, descriptive and specific about how we feel helps us to identify and acknowledge what we are experiencing and make sense of what can sometimes seem to be a whirlwind of emotions.

Whether we're feeling absolutely furious or mildly irritated, the basic emotion is anger. From grief-stricken to a bit glum, we're in the realm of sadness. Whether we're terrified beyond words or a little anxious, fear is the common denominator and from uncontainable delight to peaceful contentment we're expressing feeling happy.

So what about boredom. We so often eat because we are bored, so where does that fit in? Boredom is not exactly a feeling – but more on that later.

For now, let's take a closer look at our feelings: anger, sadness, fear and happiness.

Anger

There are many different nuances of anger – many names for it and many ways of describing it: irate, mad, annoyed, cross, vexed, irritated, indignant, irked, furious, enraged, infuriated, in a temper, incensed, raging, fuming, seething, beside oneself, choleric, outraged, sullen, surly, livid, apoplectic, hot under the collar, up in arms, foaming at the mouth, steamed up, in a lather, seeing red, sore, bent out of shape, ticked off, pissed off . . .

And so often, instead of recognising that we feel angry and finding a way to deal with it, we stuff it down with food. We numb the feeling with a bar of chocolate or a packet of crisps.

Whether we grew up in a loud, frightening home with people who shouted at us or in a quiet household where everything was 'nice' and no one ever raised their voice – or anything in between – most of us were not encouraged to feel our anger in a healthy and appropriate way and our parents and carers often did not know how to do that themselves. As a result, many of us grew up believing that anger is not ok.

We go through our daily lives swallowing our irritation, frustration and indignation. We ignore it, resist it, pretend we don't feel it, talk ourselves out of it, eat it away. None of these strategies actually deals with the anger – they just help to push it down deeper and deeper. Or we blow up constantly, shouting and being aggressive or sarcastic with the people around us and feeling guilty afterwards.

So many women ... So much anger ...

Emily has endless arguments with her husband which are invariably followed by stand-up binges in the kitchen while she feels bad about herself, bad about her eating, seething inside.

Grace sits in front of the telly on a Saturday night crunching, munching, chewing her way through a family pack of Doritos thinking about her girlfriend who is working late, again. She can't bear to admit she's furious with her and jeopardise their relationship.

Heather is late for work again. She sits on the bus churning inside. How could she be so incompetent, so useless, so unprofessional. She's *furious* with herself. How hard can it be to set the alarm and get out of the house on time? She sits there tearing off bits of croissant and angrily shoving them into her mouth.

Jane sometimes blows up at her children over something really small. She feels so tense and angry she could throttle them both . . . and then she drowns her guilt and shame with a cup of tea and a Kit Kat, and then another one, a pack of crisps and a banana.

✦

Anger is not good or bad, negative or positive. It is simply a feeling, an energy in our bodies.

We often hear people talking about negative emotions and positive emotions, good feelings and bad feelings. It's not helpful to see them in that way. How can a feeling in itself be positive or negative? It is not the feeling that is good or bad, it is what we *do* with it that makes the difference. If I scream and shout at someone or hurt and lash out when I am angry, clearly that is not a good thing. If I turn my anger on myself or squash it down under layers of resentment that could also be called negative. But if I feel angry, recognise it in myself, acknowledge it and then deal with it in a responsible, adult way without hurting or attacking anyone, how is that wrong?

We can tell ourselves that we should rise above it, that it's not helpful to feel angry, that if we don't acknowledge that we feel angry, we are not feeling it. Not so. It doesn't matter how much we resist it, the feeling won't go away on its own. In fact, the more we resist it, the bigger it gets and the harder it becomes to hold it in.

Feeling angry is normal, it's one of the many responses we have to life. It's there even when we don't feel it consciously, when we pretend we're not angry or when we stuff it down. It's there when we reason ourselves out of it. And when we ignore it or resist feeling it, it has all the power. And then, when we've swallowed one thing too many, we explode and feel furious or it leaks out in sarcastic comments and resentful jibes. It can even be a small thing that tips us over the edge. It feels like the anger is controlling us, and we are quite powerless.

Sometimes it's so uncomfortable and unfamiliar to be angry with someone that we turn the anger in on ourselves. Instead of feeling cross at the way our friend spoke to us, we eat, then we can tell ourselves that we are useless and that we deserve everything we get. We beat ourselves up because it's easier, more acceptable to be angry with ourselves than it is to be angry with someone else.

Being willing to own our anger and acknowledge it, means we can take control of it and choose how we want to express it – or not. We can take charge.

As children, when we behaved angrily, we may have been told things like:

✦ 'There's no point making a fuss, that's how it is.'

✦ 'Don't be annoyed with your sister – she didn't mean it.'

✦ 'How dare you talk to me like that?'

✦ 'One more word . . .'

✦ 'Shush, you're going to upset your mother.'

✦ 'Stop it. Stop that right now.'

✦ 'Stop being naughty!'

✦ 'Ooooh . . . look at you: temper temper, lighten up.'

The way our anger was responded to in our childhood lays down the pattern for how we manage it as adults. If you're reading this and thinking that you really never get angry, then take a close look at your sadness and your fear – the anger may be buried under those other feelings. Sometimes, tears are the only way we feel able to express our frustration and anger.

Sadness

There are so many different shades of sadness, so many ways to feel sad: unhappy, sorrowful, dejected, depressed, downcast, miserable, down, despondent, despairing, disconsolate, desolate, dismayed, wretched, glum, gloomy, doleful, dismal, melancholy, mournful, woebegone, forlorn, crestfallen, heartbroken, inconsolable, blue, down in the dumps . . .

Some of us are more comfortable feeling sad than we are feeling angry, and that appears to be particularly true of women. Somehow, feeling sad is less threatening, more manageable, more feminine. Powerful, independent women can be seen as bolshy and butch. A desperate, sad, unhappy woman is less of a threat. Other women find that for them, sadness is completely alien. They wouldn't dream of crying in front of anyone, ever.

Some of us are judgmental about sadness. We see it as weak, pathetic, useless, needy. For others, it is a useful place to hide, an ally of sorts. It is the security blanket we wrap ourselves in when things don't go the way we want or when we don't know what to do. Or perhaps we feel overwhelmed by it and however much we try to fight it, it drags us down, deeper and deeper.

Some of us talk ourselves out of feeling sad. We tell ourselves that so-and-so didn't mean to hurt our feelings, that's there's no point getting upset, that we need to put on a brave face, get through it, stiff upper lip and all that. Some of us wallow in it and only know how to comfort ourselves with food. We sit and feel sorry for ourselves with a cup of tea and the biscuit tin. Nursing our wounds with food is a well-trodden path for so many of us, maybe a lifelong habit.

So many women ... So much sadness ...

When **Alice** was twelve years old she used to sit in her dormitory at boarding school, feeling so desperately homesick. She would plough her way through her tuck box full of sweets, chocolate, biscuits and snacks. Longing for a taste of home, aching for a hug, not daring to cry.

When **Debbie's** best friend moved to another city she missed her. She missed their evenings out, bumping into her on the Broadway, popping over for a cup of tea and a piece of cake . . . cake, that's how she holds on to her. Eating cake, slice after slice. It helps her feel less heartbroken. Just for a few minutes.

Isabelle didn't shed a single tear when her grandmother died. She loved her so much and just didn't know how to let herself grieve. If she started to cry, she might never stop. She couldn't bear the pain. It was easier to pretend it wasn't there . . . and eat.

Olivia spends endless evenings at home alone, feeling down in the dumps, with just a tub of ice cream to keep her company, telling herself she'll never have anyone to share it with. She'll grow old alone, no one could possibly love her. She can completely forget herself for as long as the soothing, silky, sweetness envelops her.

✦

Food soothes our sadness or keeps us company in our moments of misery. Many of us learned that crying and feeling sad were the only way to get attention, as we'd be hugged, consoled and taken care of. While for some of us, it was quite the opposite: when we felt sad, we were met with disdain, rejection, irritation or nothing at all.

Do you ever remember being told:

✦ 'Stop crying now, that's enough. I said *stop* crying.'

✦ 'Don't be such a cry baby.'

✦ 'No use crying over spilled milk.'

✦ 'Pull yourself together.'

✦ 'Oh, for goodness sake, stop wingeing.'

✦ 'Oh, you're such a misery guts.'

✦ 'You're acting like a baby.'

✦ 'Stop feeling sorry for yourself.'

✦ 'Oh, poor you. Come here and let me make it better.'

✦ 'Oh, what's the matter? Oh, how awful, you poor thing.'

✦ 'Boo hoo, no one cares.'

As a result, many of us learned as children to avoid feeling sad because it was appropriate to protect ourselves. Or we kept coming back to it and feeling it, again and again, to get the attention we needed. Our responses as children were about survival. Our lives depended, literally *depended* on the adults around us continuing to take care of us and we adapted to make sure that they did. Whether by feeling it or avoiding it, we did whatever worked.

Today, as adults, we no longer need those mechanisms and yet we continue to behave as if we do. Today, our survival is in our hands alone. We don't have to cut ourselves off from our pain to stay alive. We don't have to cling to or wallow in our sadness to get attention. Today, it's the other way round. When we cut ourselves off from our feelings or let them overwhelm us, we are only half alive.

Feeling sad, just like feeling angry, gives us information. It's not good or bad, negative or positive. When we are willing to acknowledge that we feel sad without minimising it, talking ourselves out of it, criticising ourselves for it or wallowing in it, we can learn something of value. We can get to know parts of ourselves we didn't even know were there – strong, powerful parts that are more than capable of bearing pain, dealing with it and finding a way through it.

Fear

Just like anger and sadness, we experience fear in many different ways: terror, fright, fearfulness, horror, alarm, panic, agitation, trepidation, dread, consternation, distress, anxiety, worry, angst, unease, apprehension, nervousness, nerves, perturbation, foreboding, the creeps, the shivers, the willies, feeling jittery, twitchy, butterflies in our stomach.

There's nothing to fear

Fear is another one of those feelings which gets bad press. Fear, we are told, is weak, silly or unreasonable. We shouldn't feel afraid and, if we do, we should simply ignore our fears – conquer them, fight them, be strong, be brave.

In the excellent title of Susan Jeffers' book *Feel the Fear and Do It Anyway* the key word is *feel*. Not ignore the fear or conquer the fear – *feel* it. When we allow ourselves to acknowledge our emotions, we have a choice about where to go next, what to do, how to manage. By getting to know how we feel fear and what triggers us, we can learn to deal with it, rather than eat it away. It doesn't matter whether our fears make sense to anyone else, whether they are rational or irrational, whether they are out of proportion (in someone else's opinion) – they are there whether we want them to be or not and, by acknowledging the feeling, we can make a choice about how to feel it and begin to deal with the situations that triggered it.

So many women ... So much fear ...

Christine lives in a perpetual state of anxiety about her health. A cough becomes pneumonia, a headache could be a tumour and heartburn could be the beginnings of a heart attack. She frightens herself every day with catastrophic thoughts about falling ill and imminent death. Large bags of Haribos quieten the fear until the next twinge.

Emily remembers the sheer terror of sitting alone in the canteen at her new school and the blessed reassurance and comfort of those wonderful icing-covered doughnuts.

Leila worries that she'll never get all her work done. She puts it off with one trip after another to the fridge. Procrastinating with food. Effective and soul destroying.

Natasha is so frightened of flying that every time she boards a plane she has to have enough food in her backpack to feed an entire family. For the whole trip she eats and reads, in a vain attempt to distract herself from her fears. She fills herself up with wine gums and peanuts, sandwiches and pretzels, she drinks juice and pops in one M&M after another, reaching her destination stuffed and disgusted.

Olivia felt so nervous before an interview that she ploughed her way through a huge bag of popcorn, an entire tube of Jaffa cakes, a packet of pork scratchings and two Wagon Wheels. It was like being in a trance. She doesn't even remember the eating, just how revolting she felt afterwards and how much she hated herself.

Pam dreads going to work in the mornings. She hates her job and is petrified of her loud, obnoxious and frankly, nasty boss. She grabs a cappuccino and a croissant at the station café, then heads straight for the canteen to pick up a sausage sandwich and a couple of hash browns before she goes to her desk. Her days are punctuated with visits to the vending machine to soothe her anxiety.

✦

So many of us learned to stuff down or exaggerate our fears. When we were anxious, scared, afraid, nervous, we were told:

✦ 'Don't be silly, there's nothing to be scared of.'

✦ 'Pull yourself together.'

✦ 'I'm so worried about you.'

✦ 'You're making a mountain out of a molehill.'

✦ 'Come on, you mustn't be frightened of . . .'

✦ 'Come on now, no one likes a coward.'

✦ 'Scaredy cat, scaredy cat . . .'

✦ 'What will other people think?'

✦ 'No one else is frightened of having a go . . .'

✦ 'Be careful.'

✦ 'You're being unreasonable.'

✦ 'But sweetheart, of course monsters don't exist.'

✦ 'You're scaring me.'

It's not surprising that we continue to talk to ourselves in the same way as adults. We tell ourselves that we are stupid and ridiculous and, thankfully, our faithful friend food comes to the rescue. We can hold on to so many mixed messages: 'Don't be frightened . . .' (subtext: 'Fear is not appropriate, you shouldn't be scared'); 'Be careful' (= 'Don't do anything dangerous, *I'm* scared something will happen to you'). Paradoxically, at the same time as feeling bad about our lack of courage and assertiveness, we hold ourselves back through fear, fear of failure, fear of ridicule, fear of pain.

Fear can be a response to danger, real or perceived, large or small. It is neither good nor bad, it's how we manage it that makes the difference, that leaves us feeling in control or controlled *by* our fears. Or maybe we catastrophise – scaring ourselves with 'what-if' thinking. We panic about the things we can't control, about the future. And we create anxiety by being critical of ourselves.

When we are willing to own our fears – to recognise, explore and feel them – (without criticising ourselves for them) we have more options available to us.

Happiness

Happiness comes in many guises: cheerful, merry, joyful, carefree, untroubled, delighted, excited, in good spirits, in a good mood, lighthearted, pleased, contented, satisfied, thrilled, exhilarated, ecstatic, blissful, euphoric, overjoyed, in seventh heaven, on cloud nine, walking on air, jumping for joy, chirpy, over the moon . . .

But does happiness really lead to overeating? Are these emotions we wrestle with? Surely happy is a *good* feeling, a *positive* emotion? Why would we overeat when we're happy? It doesn't make sense. Or does it?

So many women ... So much happiness ...

Alice remembers childhood Christmases at her grandmother's, who was such a good cook. She just loved her food and would spend the whole holiday eating. It felt like one long feast and she loved every minute. Until she got home and stood on the scales.

The only way **Debbie** knows to celebrate, to treat herself or give herself a break is to eat. Preferably chocolate. Or cake. Or biscuits. It's the cheapest, easiest, loveliest way and no one else need know anything about it.

Isabelle felt so excited about going on holiday to New York for the first time that she couldn't sleep. She spent all night watching TV and eating cheese balls, peanuts, crisps – whatever she could get her hands on – and washing them down with gallons of Coke. Anything that would make the night feel less endless.

For **Natasha**, food is her pleasure, her sensuality, her luxury.
  She revels in the seductiveness of cold ice cream filling
  her mouth, the quasi ecstasy of chocolate melting on her
  tongue. She *loves* food.

◆

We tend to tell ourselves that anger, fear and sadness are the
feelings that we avoid or feel overwhelmed by. They are the feelings we think of as negative and difficult. And yet so many of us
find it as hard to let ourselves be truly happy.

Feeling anything more than quietly content is not encouraged in our society. There's something slightly shameful about
feeling too happy. Sometimes we worry that if everything really
is perfect, if we are content and happy with the way things are,
happy with what we have, then the only way is down. And it's
true that nothing stays the same for very long, so we tell ourselves that it's safer not to be too happy, better not to expect too
much, then we won't be disappointed or bereft. We stop ourselves feeling happy because we can't make it last for ever.

False modesty, constantly understating our achievements
and playing down our successes, that's the acceptable (and certainly British) way. It can be seen as somewhat crass and arro-
gant to sing our own praises, to feel too good about ourselves,
to be happy with our lives and satisfied with who we are and
what we do. It goes against the idea that we should always be
striving to do better, push ourselves harder, achieve more and
think of others before ourselves. How can we really be content
when we are so imperfect? What would people think? And if
we are happy and they are not, isn't that rubbing their noses in
it, uncaring and unkind?

And if we are really happy, if we like ourselves or – dare we say it – love ourselves, will those we care about still love *us*? Or will they reject us? How will they react if we are no longer needy or weak or lost?

So often we are brought up with values and beliefs that stop us from reaching our full potential. Of course, that is very rarely our parents' intention. They don't do it on purpose. Often, they are simply passing on patterns and behaviours that were handed down to them by their own parents and grandparents. There is nothing to be gained from blaming them and everything to be gained from acknowledging that as adults, we are free to choose what we believe and how we behave. And we don't have to keep looking to the future for our source of happiness.

As a child, do you ever remember hearing:

✦ 'Don't get too excited . . . you'll only end up disappointed.'

✦ 'Don't count your chickens before they hatch.'

✦ 'Shush' (to a happy, bouncy, excited child) ' . . . tone it down a bit, will you.'

✦ 'Stop boasting, nobody likes a big head.'

✦ In a school report: 'Could do better.'

✦ To a child who finds school easy and fun: 'Just wait till you get to secondary school, you'll have to work much harder then.'

✦ 'Life's not just one big party you know.'

✦ 'Stop showing off; not everyone's as lucky as you.'

✦ 'Shush, you're making a scene.'

✦ 'She's so full of herself.'

✦ 'Wipe that smile off your face.'

✦ 'What have you got to be so chirpy about?'

It's not surprising that we tone ourselves down, keep ourselves from being too happy, too big, too full. And by not expressing ourselves, by not allowing ourselves to feel good, happy, excited or ecstatic, we end up feeling low and depressed. If we constantly parrot those unhelpful phrases to ourselves to keep ourselves small, often we eat and eat and that's when we get big.

Food and celebrations

Of course, we are not all miserable and grumpy all the time. There are many ways in which we do let ourselves feel happy. And then, very often, in our joys and celebrations, food plays a significant part.

Food has become almost synonymous with festivities. When we have something to celebrate, we do it with food. And there's nothing wrong with that. Food is one of the joys of life. If we allow it to be. When we let go of the guilt, we can allow ourselves to enjoy food for what it is: a delicious, sensuous, nourishing pleasure.

And yet, many a time we eat just because it's the done thing. We use celebrations as an *excuse* to eat. We spend so much time depriving ourselves of the foods we love that any happy moment is a good reason to eat cake, chocolate, have a proper sit-down three-course meal or a gargantuan buffet. A celebration turns into an excuse to indulge, to overdo it, to eat till we feel we could burst. We keep eating long after we stop being hungry.

For some of us, food is one of the few, sometimes the only, route to pleasure. We can rely on food to be there, to provide us with a moment of abandon and gratification. It may only be fleeting and we may regret it every time, but we soon forget and return to the promise of pleasure.

By exploring how food and happiness are intertwined, you will have more choices available to you and you won't always turn to food in happy times.

BOREDOM

We've included boredom in this chapter because so many women say they eat when they are *feeling* bored. Yet boredom is not really a feeling. What exactly *is* boredom? One definition is: feeling weary because one is unoccupied or lacks interest in one's current activity. The question is, what *feelings* do we experience when we have nothing to do or when we are not interested in or enjoying what we are doing?

Do we feel sad, miserable, low, dejected, depressed? Do we feel afraid, anxious, worried, nervous? Do we feel angry, annoyed, pissed off, frustrated?

So many of us seek to avoid *feeling* at all costs. Instead, we fill every moment, staying occupied, avoiding pain, anguish, excitement, discomfort, filling ourselves up with food.

So many women ... So much boredom ...

Fatima is stuck in her room revising for exams which are looming. Biology . . . yawn. English . . . yawn. History . . . triple yawn. She's so bored that only a constant stream of peanuts and Coke keeps her from falling asleep at her desk. At least her father is leaving her alone because he doesn't want to interrupt her 'concentration' and she can eat away from his prying eyes.

Grace is spending an evening in front of the telly. Bored. Bored. Bored. The only activity is her regular trips to the kitchen to find something to eat. Anything to give herself a bit of respite from the utter boredom.

Heather is staring at her screen. She's at the office and there are still hours to go before she can pack up and go home. She is soooo bored. She's just finished a cup of coffee. A trip to the vending machine will waste a few more minutes. What will it be this time? Crisps? A Kit Kat?

Isabelle remembers being at home in the holidays, her mum out at work, watching James Bond movies with her sister, one after the other, over and over again. They ate anything they could get their hands on, all day, to while away the tedium. Even now, she can't watch a film without eating something.

Jane at nap time. Stuck at home, alone, with nothing to do. Or at least, nothing she feels like doing. Picking at leftovers in the fridge, lasagna, baked beans, trifle, whatever is there. It helps her numb the desperate boredom . . . day after day, despite her daily promises to resist, her resolve to do something useful . . . tomorrow.

✦

There *are* other ways besides eating to respond to boredom, to emptiness, to the discomfort of having nothing to do. Yet food is so very often the filler of choice. Eating gives us something to focus on when we don't know what else to do. Eating gives us a way of punctuating an uneventful day, creating comforting breaks, giving ourselves a treat, something to look forward to. Eating ensures we are never just left alone with ourselves.

Do you ever remember being told:

✦ 'If you're bored, think of something to do.'

✦ 'Well do something then.'

✦ 'You've got plenty of toys and things to do, just get on with it.'

✦ 'Only boring people get bored.'

Some of us are terrified of boredom, while others think that it says something about us – that if we are not *doing*, we *are* nothing. Either way, we are desperate to fill the empty moments. We are hell-bent on *not* experiencing boredom.

What would it have been like if our parents or teachers had just let us be when we were bored, shrugged their shoulders knowingly, with a kind smile and trusted that we would, when we were ready, move from boredom to something else. It's not surprising that we have a low tolerance level for boredom.

TAKE ACTION

The next time you overeat, tune in to your feelings. This isn't a long, drawn-out, protracted affair. Tuning in takes a matter of seconds (or maybe a little longer to begin with, but certainly no more than a minute). And when you've tuned in once, plan to do it again. And again. Often.

→

You can tune in to your feelings at random times during your day. Practise – the more you do it, the better.

Tips for tuning in to your feelings

- Find one word in the angry, sad, afraid, happy spectrum that fits how you feel in that precise instant.

- You don't need to go into a story about it, to justify or explain it. And you don't even need to understand it. Your job is to notice it with curiosity, and name it.

- You don't have to do anything with it. You don't have to feel it or express it or fix it. Just name it.

- To begin with, you may not have a clue how you feel. We spend so many years being told how we ought to feel or what not to feel that we forget how to identify our feelings. Keep on tuning in, it will come.

- If you tune in and are feeling a myriad emotions all at once, see if you can narrow it down to just one: which is the strongest?

- If you're finding it a challenge to put a name to how you are feeling, you might like to use the words listed below to inspire you.

Happy
Happy Content Pleased Glad Joyful Cheerful Blissful Excited Ecstatic Delighted

→

Angry

Angry Annoyed Irritated Livid Furious Enraged Infuriated Outraged Cross Irate Sullen

Sad

Sad Gloomy Miserable Cheerless Unhappy Glum Dismal Morose Melancholy

Afraid

Afraid Frightened Fearful Anxious Scared Terrified Nervous Worried Alarmed Panicky

If you struggle with remembering to tune in to your feelings, find an effective way to remind or prompt yourself: your screen saver, Post-it notes, a note in your diary, a reminder on your phone.

What if I feel nothing much?

Don't let yourself off the hook. We are always feeling *something*. If you keep on coming up with 'feeling ok' or 'nothing much' or 'numb', it might be an indication that you're not ready to go there right now. And that's ok. The important thing is to acknowledge that at this point in time you're not yet ready to name your feeling. Give yourself time and keep coming back to this exercise. Sometimes, bringing feelings into the open can feel scary. It's like opening a can of worms: we don't know what we'll have to deal with and, as we said before, that's quite often why we overeat in the first place.

YOUR **ACTION** CHECKLIST

☐ **Make it official**: call it overeating

☐ **Observe yourself with curiosity**: overeat with awareness

☐ **Identify your triggers**: find out why you overeat

☐ **Lighten the load**: talk about what it's really like

☐ **Find out about your forbidden foods**: make a list

☐ **Tune in to your Gremlin**: get to know it

☐ **Tune in to your feelings**: name and acknowledge them

CHAPTER **EIGHT**

•

The Overeating Body

IN THE TWO PREVIOUS CHAPTERS, we have seen how our Gremlins and our feelings can take over and drive us to overeat. In this chapter, we'll be showing you how we embody those thoughts and feelings. Whatever we are thinking and feeling, we do it with our whole body: our breathing, our posture, every muscle, every limb, every part of our body is involved.

Everyone has an overeating body. Most of us are so cut off from our physical selves that we have no idea what's going on in our bodies, which is ironic, given that most of us spend so much time and energy trying to change them. The aim of this chapter is to tune in and to reconnect with our bodies, so that we recognise the part they play in our overeating.

Let's start by looking at how body talk can impact both our thoughts and our feelings: when we are in charge of our feelings, our thoughts *and* our bodies, rather than at their mercy, we are also in charge of our eating.

SO MANY WOMEN ... SO MANY OVEREATING BODIES ...

It's time to reconnect with the physical, with the part of us that embodies or acts out our thoughts and our feelings and actually does the overeating. It's time to meet the overeating body ...

Alice has had another long stressful day at work. She pops into the supermarket on her way home to grab something for dinner and walks out with a bag stuffed full of all her favourite binge foods. Now she's standing at the counter, still in her coat, doughnut in hand, about to take a bite.

Body talk: tensing her neck, pulling her shoulders forward, sweaty palms, brick-like sensation in her belly, breathing fast.

Becky is having dinner with friends. The conversation is flowing, the atmosphere is relaxed, the food is delicious. She's looking at the pudding menu, trying to decide what to have, thinking she really shouldn't . . .

Body talk: belly straining against her tight waistband, sitting slumped in chair, arms and legs heavy, turning her mouth down, fixing her gaze on the menu, breathing very slowly and shallowly.

Christine is in Starbucks. It's her lunch break. She's only got fifteen minutes before her next patient. She's sitting on a bar stool, staring out of the window, mechanically alternating sips of caramel latte and bites of chocolate muffin.

Body talk: stiff all over, gnawing in the pit of her stomach, jutting out her bottom jaw, frowning.

Debbie is standing in the queue to pay at the petrol station with two Galaxy bars in her hand.

Body talk: constricted sensation in her throat, turning her mouth down, her gaze fixed, slumping her shoulders, teary.

Emily is sitting in the car, in the Sainsbury's car park looking at the pack of cocktail sausages on her lap.

Body talk: breathing shallowly, flushed cheeks, clenching her teeth, flaring her nostrils, tightening her muscles.

Fatima is ravenous. It's midnight and she's standing in front of the fridge about to eat.

Body talk: opening her eyes wide, breathing very quickly, shaking all over, throbbing temples.

Grace is alone at home in front of the telly having passed up yet another invitation to go out to dinner with friends. She's just come back from the kitchen with a third packet of Doritos. She's sitting on the sofa with the pack in one hand and the remote in the other.

Body talk: bloated, dry mouth, narrowing her eyes, biting her lip, twitching her foot.

Heather is at the wheel of her car, waiting in the queue at the Drive-Thru for another late-night fast-food fest.

Body talk: thighs, belly, chest and arms constricted by her tight clothes, skin pressing into the fabric, hyperventilating, hands clutching the steering wheel, hunching her shoulders, holding her breath.

Isabelle is at home on a Saturday afternoon. Home alone. She's bored out of her mind and there's no one on Facebook. She's standing in front of the food cupboard, trying to decide what else to eat.

Body talk: drumming her fingers, curling her toes, rubbing her lips together hard, clenching her buttocks.

Jane is clearing the table. As she ferries plates over to the dishwasher she is eating what's left on all of them. It's been another endless day.

Body talk: everything aching, heavy arms, heavy legs, chapped lips, pounding at the back of her head, breathing irregularly, shallowly.

Kate is having Sunday lunch at her mum's after three weeks of no carbs. She's staring at a Yorkshire pudding.

Body talk: salivating, sitting forward on her seat, breathing through her mouth, pressing her knees together, sitting on her hands.

Leila is sitting at her desk in between trips to the fridge. There are 130 emails in her inbox and sixteen items on her to-do list. She'll never get it all done. She distracts herself by thinking about what to eat next.

Body talk: dragging sensation in her chest, blinking a lot, chewing her fingers, sighing, crossing her legs, tapping her foot.

Natasha is at home with friends, playing a board game. They're having a real laugh and one of her friends has brought her absolute favourite: carrot cake with thick cream cheese frosting. She's been back for seconds and wants more.

Body talk: warm beads of sweat on her forehead, heart racing, limbs soft and loose, laughing.

Olivia is at her sister's wedding sitting at the top table, wishing she were anywhere else. She gets up and heads for the wedding cake.

Body talk: hot, sweating, clothes too tight, hunching her shoulders, staring down at the floor, breathing slowly, skin itchy all over.

Pam is at the office. Someone has brought in some fairy cakes to celebrate their birthday and is handing them round. Pam is still stuffed from lunch, but she can't bear to say no.

Body talk: stomach stretched and uncomfortable pressing against her waistband, fiddling with her pen, frowning, grinding her teeth.

TUNING IN TO YOUR OVEREATING BODY

We feel our emotions with our whole body. We think with our whole body. In fact, everything we do and experience in life, we do with our whole body. We *are* our bodies, despite the fact that sometimes we behave as if they are independent entities. Something we *have* rather than something we *are*.

Tuning in to our overeating body is a bit like tuning in to our feelings and our Gremlins (see Chapters 6 and 7). It's about focusing on what we are doing, how we are holding and shaping our bodies, so that we become aware of ourselves, rather than behaving unconsciously.

Let's do a quick experiment. Think of something you feel annoyed about – a person or situation you are irritated with. Take a moment to come up with something; it doesn't have to be a big thing, just any situation or person you are annoyed about. Now think about it for a few seconds. See it as a picture in your mind's eye, if that helps. Really focus on *feeling* annoyed – you won't have to feel it for long, just for a minute. As you do that, tune in to what you are doing with the different parts of your body. How are you *embodying* feeling annoyed? How is your body *being* annoyed?

Pay attention to your **breathing.** Are you aware of breathing:

shallowly	quickly	up in your chest
deeply	slowly	down into your belly
hyperventilating	unevenly	holding your breath

Now move on to your **posture**. How are you holding your body? Are you aware of:

leaning forward

leaning back

slumping

being rigid

Now focus on each **body part** in turn. Your feet, calves, thighs, buttocks, hips, abdomen, chest, arms, hands, shoulders, back, neck. Are you aware of doing any of the following:

jiggling	scratching	arching
tapping	tugging	releasing
curling	straining	picking
bouncing	clutching	pins & needles
clenching	tensing	numbness
twiddling	relaxing	tightening
loosening	rubbing	releasing
throbbing		drumming
squeezing		

Now, hold that feeling of annoyance for a bit longer, keep thinking about that situation or person you feel annoyed with, just a few more seconds and focus on your **face**: your mouth, eyes, jaw, cheeks, lips, teeth, etc. Are you aware of:

pursing	staring	squeezing
pinching	gazing	pouting
grinding	blinking	laughing
biting	tearing	smiling
nibbling	flushing	grinning
chewing	widening	frowning
flaring	narrowing	twitching
tensing	aching	sniffing
swallowing		

Next, focus on the sensations **inside** your body. What sensations are you aware of in your head and your throat? Are you aware of how your heart is beating? What sensations can you feel in your stomach, your belly?

How do you feel in your **clothes**? Are you aware of any tightness or itching? Just pay attention to any sensations you become aware of.

Ok. You can stop thinking about the annoying situation now, you can stop feeling annoyed! What did you find out? How do you embody feeling annoyed? What does your annoyed body look like?

WE EMBODY OUR THOUGHTS AND FEELINGS

The fascinating thing is that it works both ways. When we think about something and have a feeling about it, we embody that emotion, physically, with every part of our bodies, as you just experienced if you did the experiment just now. And on the flip side, the way we hold and shape our bodies can *create* or sustain our feelings: we impact how we feel by what we are doing with our bodies.

Take your annoyed body. Let's say that when you tuned in just now, you became aware of breathing very shallowly, of slightly tensing almost every muscle in your body, of being very still, of clenching your jaw, of staring straight ahead of you, of frowning and tightening your mouth, of drawing your fingers in towards your palms, of pulling your belly in a bit . . . (You may well have embodied your annoyed feelings very differently, we each have our unique ways of doing it, so – we're just using this as an example). When you become practised at tuning in to your body, at recognising that this is how your body is creating 'annoyed' for example, you can experiment with changing the way you are holding yourself and in doing so, you will change the way you feel too.

But we're running away with ourselves. We don't want to change anything just yet. Awareness is the first step. Without knowing what we do, we can't choose to do something different. So practising tuning in and becoming aware of your body will give you all the information you need to make changes, when you are ready. The more you find out about your overeating body, the better equipped you will be to stop overeating.

TAKE ACTION

Tune in to your overeating body. Aim to tune in at any point when you overeat. When you've done it once, plan to do it again. And again. You can tune in to your body at random times during your day, just as we suggested you do with your Gremlin and feelings. Practise – the more you do it, the better.

Tips for tuning in to your overeating body

Describe what you are doing with your body, anything that you are aware of. Scan your:

- breathing
- posture
- body parts

→

- face
- internal sensations
- clothes
- skin.

You don't have to *do* anything with this information for now. You don't have to change anything. Just keep tuning in and describe whatever you notice. Your aim is awareness.

YOUR **ACTION** CHECKLIST

☐ **Make it official**: call it overeating

☐ **Observe yourself with curiosity:** overeat with awareness

☐ **Identify your triggers:** find out why you overeat

☐ **Lighten the load:** talk about what it's really like

☐ **Find out about your forbidden foods:** make a list

☐ **Tune in to your Gremlin:** get to know it

☐ **Tune in to your feelings**: name and acknowledge them

☐ **Tune in to your overeating body:** listen to your body talk

CHAPTER **NINE**

•

The Pause

YOUR INVESTIGATIONS ARE nearly over. In this chapter, we're going to use everything you've learned so far to take another step towards stopping overeating. We are going to introduce you to **The Pause**. Pausing is nothing more than delaying or interrupting your overeating for a maximum of sixty seconds, so that you can tune in to your thoughts, your feelings and your body talk all at the same time.

Pausing serves two purposes. The first is to start getting used to interrupting the often unconscious and automatic hand-to-mouth action that takes place when we overeat. The second purpose of The Pause is to allow you to tune in to and discover the interconnection between your thoughts your feelings and your body talk.

If you are still not absolutely clear about who or what your Gremlin is – if, despite tuning in, you haven't really heard it or identified a dialogue, as such – pausing will be doubly help-ful. Because if the Gremlin thinks, even for just a few seconds, that there's a chance that you won't eat, it will show itself in an attempt to persuade you, to make sure that you do. This is particularly true for those of us who overeat, as if on automatic pilot: the kind of overeating where there seems to be no real dialogue, where the Gremlin is silent or elusive. The Pause will tease it out.

PAUSING: AN OPPORTUNITY TO TUNE IN

Pausing is not about putting off eating, holding on until the minute has past and you can finally just eat. Pausing is about tuning in and experimenting with not overeating, just for a minute. That's how we find out what it's like to do something different, to change a behaviour – by practising it, experimenting with it, experiencing it, playing with it. One step at a time. Gradually. Pausing is a stepping stone towards stopping.

As you have been tuning in to your thoughts, your feelings and your body talk, you may already have discovered for yourself how they are connected. The way you think and what you tell yourself (aka your Gremlin) produces feelings, and what you feel produces a physical response. Or, another way to look at it is that you embody your feelings; you hold a shape, a body form, which then generates or sustains a feeling.

So our thinking, our feelings and our body talk are all interlinked, all interdependent.

SO MANY WOMEN ... PAUSING ...

As always, we have our friends to show us how it's done.

Alice: God, this is good, I love Nutella. I could pause. Can I do it? I *could*. I can't. No way. I need this. Mmmm . . . That's better. I'm not ready. This is such a tricky time of day. I've picked the most difficult. I *will* pause tomorrow at work.

Becky: Just a forkful of pasta left. I'm going to put the fork down and pause. Quick, set the timer on my phone. Sixty seconds, tune in. Ok, thoughts: what am I thinking? 'I really want it. I really want it.' God, there it is, that's my Gremlin. But I *do* really want it. I *can't* leave it. What am I feeling? What am I feeling? Longing, longing, longing for more pasta. What about my body? Um, mouth full of saliva? I don't know what the connection is . . . um . . . Beep beep beep.

Christine: At the cinema with a bucket of popcorn. Bucket – mouth. Bucket – mouth. Bucket – mouth. I could pau . . . Bucket – mouth. Munch, munch. I don't want to stop. I don't even want to pause. I like this. Bucket – mouth. Munch, munch. Wait. What if I stop, just this once? No, not stop, just pause. Yeah, and sit here in the dark, like a wally? Yes, like a wally. Ok, so what am I thinking? Nothing really, except EAT. That's all I can think of. It's that bloody autopilot thing again. Feeling? Well, pissed off now, but nothing much before. Well actually, I suppose happy with the popcorn. Body talk? I'm pretty rigid . . . tense all over. I suppose I sort of become a robot. Makes sense. Oh! That's interesting . . .

Debbie: Oh God, I'm hopeless. Here I go again. (Sees a Post-it note with the word 'Pause!' written on it.) I said I'd do it today. No, I can't, I can't – I just can't. What's the point, anyway? Yes, I *can*. It's just for a minute. Maybe just half a minute. It's ok. I can tune in for just thirty seconds. Ok. What am I thinking? Look at it all. Why do I do this to myself. Why? I'm so out of control. Why can't I be normal? Hold on, is that what I'm thinking? Is this my Gremlin? It is. It's my worn-out moaner. This is exciting! How am I feeling? Ok now. Ok. I'm feeling ok. What about my body? Tingly. I'm feeling all tingly.

Emily: God, that sausage roll looks good. I'll eat it on the way home. Oh, but I said I'd pause today. This is it. Now what? Pause. Pause. Pause. Breathe. I'm meant to be tuning in. Fuck this. I want the sausage roll.

Fatima: I think everyone's in bed now. (Opens the fridge.) Mum's trifle. Shall I get a spoon? Ok, ok, I'll get a spoon in a minute. I'll do the pause thing. Just for a minute. Oven clock. Ok. Shit, what if someone walks in? What if *Dad* walks in? What am I telling myself? I'm pathetic. I feel sick. This is so awful. I don't even really want it, but it's so unfair, I had to sit there with my bloody apple while they all had trifle. God, that's all true. I'm feeing . . . terrified. But all that *is* scary. Oh shit, that's terrible. I'm so tense, and I'm hardly breathing. I feel like crying.

Grace: I can't believe Megan's working late again. What did I do wrong this time? What's on telly? Is there any of that Ben & Jerry's left? Right, one scoop . . . no, two scoops, caramel sauce, sprinkles. Let's do this properly. Get comfy on the couch. Where's the remote? Hang on. Hang on. I can

do the pause thing. Nah, it's going to melt. Too sad, too
pissed off, too lonely. Hang on, hang on, that's a feeling!
Uh-huh, it's lots of feelings. Which is it, then? Ok, lonely
isn't a feeling, it's a fact. So that leaves sad and pissed off.
I don't know. Am I more sad or more pissed off. Pissed off,
actually. God! *Really* pissed off. Why did I think I was sad,
then? Fuck. I'm confused now. Can you feel sad *and* pissed
off? Well wait, what was I thinking about? I was wondering
why Megan didn't want to be at home with me – what I'd
done wrong. I suppose that makes me sad. But then it also
makes me angry. Yes. Angry. Wow. Oh . . . the ice cream's
melting . . .

Heather: Wait. Look at it. Pause, go on, just this once. Please.
Oh stop it. This is ridiculous. You are ridiculous. Pathetic.
Do you really think that book is going to make any
difference? Look at yourself, sitting in a car park in the dark,
like some weirdo. Some fat weirdo. Just eat it you greedy
pig, stop being so pathetic. No, wait . . . you're that devil.
Stop it, please. Don't you want me to get better? Better at
what, you stupid cow? It won't work for you. Look at how
fucked up you are.

Isabelle: (At her desk, chewing a pencil.) I wish I could go out.
I'm so bored. What can I eat? I'll go down and see. Delay it
for a minute? Er, ok. I'll never be able to stop this though. I
know I won't. I've tried so many things before. It all sounds
ok, and I liked the book, but I just don't think I can do it.
I need something more. Maybe I need professional help.
Maybe I am one of those hopeless cases that no one can
help . . . How long now? Twenty-three seconds. I wonder if
what I was thinking just then was my Gremlin? Well, what am

I supposed to do with it now? Just notice. That's what it says.
Well I've noticed and it wasn't very uplifting.

Jane: Oh God, I'm tired. I'm sooooo tired. Ok, I'll just have
this and get back to the laundry before the baby wakes
up. (Sitting at the table with a cup of tea and the biscuit tin
open in front of her.) Ahhhh! That's good. I can't believe
how exhausted I am. I literally can't stand up. I'm hurting
everywhere. My back is killing me. And my legs . . . my legs!
What've I done to my neck? I can't turn it this way anymore.
Oh bugger. Is this body talk? I suppose it is. Ok, what else
is going on? I want a biscuit. I *so* want a biscuit. Is that my
Gremlin? It's not saying much, is it? What about feelings?
What am I feeling? Fed up really. Yes, tired, fed up and
wanting a biscuit – that's a pretty accurate reading. Ah! I've
paused and tuned in!

Kate: Right. Where did I save that worksheet? Oh, there it
is. Right. Tune in to thoughts: I'm telling myself I might as
well eat it now because I'm going to in the end, anyway.
Tune in to feelings. No idea. Right, look at the sheet it's got
the words on it. Worried? No, not worried. Nervous? Yes,
nervous is good. Right. Body talk. Scan . . . scan . . . what's
going on? Oh, I'm biting my cheek. Ow, that hurts. My neck
is killing me. I'm not surprised – I'm all tensed up and tight.
Right. Done. That wasn't so bad. I can eat now. Oh.

Leila: Cup of tea, biscuit tin. Hobnobs, yesss! No, hang on.
I'm supposed to be pausing. Ok. Deep breath. Here goes.
Mmm . . . Tune in. So, first it's thoughts. What am I thinking?
Well now I'm thinking about what I'm thinking! That's silly.
What was I thinking just before. I know. I was thinking about

all those bloody emails. I was telling myself I'll never get through them. I was fretting. That's an old-fashioned word; Mum would have said that. Anyway, yeah – that makes sense: if I was worrying about not getting through all my emails, I suppose that's how I was making myself fret . . . How funny. This is ok actually. Ok, next: body. God, my shoulders ache. Not surprising since they're right up by my ears. Mmm . . . Hobnobs . . . I suppose I could put them back. I'm not really hungry. I'll have them later, when I am. No big deal. That was easy. I can do that again, definitely.

Natasha: This is nice. Good food, good friends. What shall I try next? Mmmm . . . spring rolls. Nat, put the chopsticks down. Do it now. Come on, you promised you'd pause tonight. Just once. Oh gawd, there are only two left. What if they go and I don't get one? Just tune in. My legs feel so tense and my bum. It feels like I'm pulling my stomach in. And I'm not breathing very much. My heart's beating like the clappers. I'm worrying. I'm worrying that there won't be enough food for me . . . I can't do this here. Loo. I'll go to the loo. (In the loo.) Deep breath. What about my Gremlin? She was having a field day. It's like nothing matters, like I just want to enjoy myself. I don't care. I don't want to stop. Why should I, anyway? I love Chinese food and so what if I eat a few too many spring rolls? So what if I'm stuffed? It's hardly the end of the world. I think that's my Gremlin talking. Because I *should* stop eating now, really. That was way more than a minute.

Olivia: I promised. I promised I'd practise pausing today. No, I can't do this. I'm terrified. Ok, that's a start. I'm terrified. Why am I terrified? I don't know . . . I don't know. Breath. I'm not breathing. I'm terrified because I'm telling myself that this is my last chance. That if this doesn't work, I'll just go on eating for ever. That I'm not good enough to see it through. That's what I tell myself all the time . . . about everything. But it's true, I'm not good enough. I *can't* do this. I just can't. Well, I can. I just paused. I'm still feeling terrified, but I did just pause. Maybe I can do this. Maybe I can.

Pam: Mmmm, I might have another one, otherwise they'll just go to waste. No. I'm going to buckle down and tune in this time. I've got to. At least once, otherwise what's the point of spending money on a book. I mean really, I could've borrowed it from the library. Oh! Hello, Granny. Right, tuning in. Well the Gremlin bit is pretty easy: waste not, want not and all that. Ok, on to feelings: anxious, I suppose. Anxious at the thought of wasting food. Ahhhhh! So that's how it works. Body? Bloated. I feel bloated. I always feel bloated. It must be my period. Or maybe it's because I eat too much . . .

THERE'S NO RIGHT WAY TO PAUSE

We all pause and tune in in different ways.

For many of us it starts with catching our Gremlin. We're good at recognising our thoughts and hearing how we talk to ourselves. As women, we spend a lot of time *thinking* about our eating. So it's no surprise that tuning in to our thinking can be quite easy. For some of us, it's our emotions that are often at the forefront. We feel and feel and feel. When we tune in, the first thing that hits us is the feeling. And for a few, it's our body we are most tuned in to. We know our physical selves very well, using our bodies as a barometer.

So when you're pausing and tuning in, go with the flow. Whatever you become aware of first, let that be the starting point. And then tune in to the other two. If you find any one component particularly challenging, keep practising, you will get there.

TAKING YOUR TIME

In the next section of this book, we're going to show you how to manage your Gremlin, your feelings and your body talk to achieve a different outcome, so that you don't have to eat to deal with them.

For now, the focus is on bringing all three together, learning as much as possible about how they are connected and how they impact each other. For some of us, this comes easily and we are willing to have a go. It doesn't feel like a big deal and the more we do it, the easier it gets. And for others, it takes a lot of effort. We want to, but we resist, rebel or even just forget. We think about pausing, but don't do it.

Stay with it. Keep reminding yourself that it's an option and when you are ready, you'll do it. It can take a while to be willing to take the plunge, and eventually you will.

TAKE ACTION

Pause just for one minute and tune in. Tune in to your **thoughts**; see if you can identify what your Gremlin is saying. Tune in to your **feelings** and tune in to your **body talk**.

→

Pause either before you overeat and delay it for sixty seconds or interrupt yourself while you're eating – either as soon you remember or can manage.

Make sure The Pause really is just sixty seconds at most. Find a way of timing it. It's important to give yourself a time limit, so that you know that there will be an end to it.

If you find this step tricky, if you find yourself rebelling, resisting, thinking about it and just not doing it, that's fine. Be aware of your resistance or reluctance and, when you are ready, take yourself gently by the hand and have a go. Tell yourself that you will do it *once*. Just this once, to see what it's like. You are not promising to pause every single time you eat. Would you be willing to have a go, just once?

Pausing, not eating straight away, even if it's just for one minute, *will* have a consequence. It will produce a response of some kind – a feeling, a Gremlin, a bodily response . . . something. Keep tuning in.

A step-by-step guide to pausing

Step 1 Make a decision to **pause**.

Step 2 Set your timer, look at the clock.

Step 3 Delay or interrupt your eating for a maximum of sixty seconds.

Step 4 Tune in.

Step 5 After sixty seconds, eat (or not).

Step 6 Appreciate yourself for pausing.

Step 7 Plan to do it again.

Don't stop overeating

Remember, the idea is not to *stop* overeating altogether just yet. For now, the aim is for you to pause and tune in and find out as much as you can about your overeating: about your Gremlin, your feelings and your body talk and how all of that ties up. Pausing is also an experiment – you're giving yourself just a minute to experience what it might be like not to overeat. Of course, if in the process, you realise you'd rather not overeat, then that's fine; you don't have to *force* yourself! And when you do overeat, do so with awareness.

YOUR **ACTION** CHECKLIST

☐ **Make it official**: call it overeating

☐ **Observe yourself with curiosity:** overeat with awareness

☐ **Identify your triggers**: find out why you overeat

→

☐ **Lighten the load:** talk about what it's really like

☐ **Find out about your forbidden foods:** make a list

☐ **Tune in to your Gremlin:** get to know it

☐ **Tune in to your feelings**: name and acknowledge them

☐ **Tune in to your overeating body:** listen to your body talk

☐ **Pause:** for just one minute

Go!

IT'S TIME TO USE EVERYTHING you have learned to *stop* overeating.

If you've been experimenting with the action ideas in the previous chapters, you'll have lots of experience of tuning in. As a result, you'll be aware of how your Gremlin operates, what you are feeling and what you do with your body. You'll also have had several opportunities to pause – to experiment with what it's like to stop overeating, if only for a minute. So, armed with this knowledge and experience, you're ready to **GO**. It's finally time.

If you've skipped straight to this section, or if you've decided to read the whole book before taking any action, go right back to the beginning and work through the actions at the end of each chapter. If you try stopping without having done the groundwork, it won't work. And if you've been experimenting and you don't feel ready to move to on to this next stage, that's fine too. Stick with the actions in the STEADY chapters until you're ready.

In Chapter 10, 'Embrace Temptation', we'll be inviting you to do just that and allow your forbidden foods into your life, officially. Bear with us, you'll soon discover how this is the only way to stop craving and overeating them. And it gets better, because in Chapter 11, we'll reveal 'The Overeater's Secret Superpowers'. Yes, really, Superpowers.

→

With these tools under your belt you will be invincible.

But don't take our word for it – as ever Alice, Becky, Christine and the others will show you how to take action and make it happen.

So, ready, steady, **GO!**

CHAPTER **TEN**

•

Embrace Temptation

As you've probably discovered by now, much of the overeating we do has nothing to do with the food itself. Our Gremlins tend not to be particularly fussy eaters, pretty much anything will do. It doesn't matter *what* we are overeating: cake, soup, crisps, cereal bars, chocolate, yoghurt . . . they'll even settle for carrot sticks, if that's the only thing available. There are times, however, when we seem inexorably drawn to specific foods. Only they will do. We crave them, try to resist them and end up giving in and overeating them. These invariably feature on a forbidden-food list because we label them bad, naughty, off limits, even dangerous. We do our best to resist temptation. We try really hard not to eat them or to eat them only in moderation. And yet, these are so often the very foods we end up overeating. Despite our best intentions, resistance is futile.

In this chapter, we'll be explaining how to turn your forbidden foods into just ordinary foods. The best way we know to do that, to stop craving and overeating them, is to stop them being forbidden and to embrace temptation. When you can walk past salami, chocolate cake, chips, takeaways, burgers, etc. with a 'Yeah, and?' shrug, imagine how different your life will be.

NORMALISING FORBIDDEN FOODS

What would it be like not to deprive yourself of anything; for *any* reason. By legalising your forbidden foods you take away the magic power they seem to hold over you. By eating them whenever you want them, they stop being special and become normal. Imagine replacing the fruit in your fruit bowl with a pile of chocolate bars or a mountain of peanuts. What would it be like if you could have one or a handful every time you felt like it? When was the last time you walked past the apples and the oranges and couldn't resist? (Of course, if you have ever been on a low-carb diet, you may well have found yourself salivating in front of the fruit bowl; no surprise, since they *were* forbidden.) If our forbidden foods are there all the time, and we can have them whenever we want, they become ordinary. No big deal. Eventually, we stop even noticing that they are there.

This may seem to go against your principles, ethics or beliefs and fly in the face of weight-loss and healthy-eating guidelines. The fact is, you are probably eating these foods anyway. Often, more of them than you need and far more than you would eat if they were allowed.

We eat these foods anyway, usually in secret or hoping nobody will notice, usually feeling ashamed and guilty and beating ourselves up and often with little real enjoyment. Legalising them and having them when you want them will free you to make real *choices* and ironically, in the long term, you are likely to eat less of them than when they were off limits.

AM I ADDICTED?

So what about the claims that certain foods are addictive and *that's* the real reason we overeat them? That we are powerless to stop because of a physiological reaction in our bodies. And what about the idea that some of the artificial additives in foods are designed to *make* us overeat?

All that might be true. The way we see it is this: *you* are the only person who can find out whether that holds true for you. Rather than taking someone else's word for it, how would it be to find out for yourself?

By tuning in and experimenting with the suggestions in this book, you'll be in a position to find out. You'll know from first-hand experience what happens to your body and your appetite when you eat sugar or wheat or dairy (or whatever food it is). You'll then be able to make decisions about what to eat – not based on scientific evidence, which may or may not apply to you, not based on the suggestion of a doctor or 'specialist' or author or friend – based on *your own experience*, which we believe is indisputable. All of us are different and have a unique response to what we eat. You are the only reliable benchmark.

FOOD IS NOT A DRUG

So what do you do if, as you experiment, you discover that you do have a physical response to eating certain foods? You may find that when you eat sugar or wheat or any other food, it feels like you cannot stop. Then what? You could stop eating those foods altogether. It is tempting to think that by eliminating them from your diet, rather than legalising them, you will eliminate the problem all together. Like alcoholics do with alcohol. You could decide never to eat white flour or sugar again. Ever. Like you might decide never to have another drink, if you were an alcoholic. That definitely works for alcoholics. In fact, it's the only way: to stop drinking alcohol altogether. One day at a time. But does it work for food?

It sounds simple enough and yet wheat and sugar are not drugs: they are not illegal, you don't have to be a certain age to buy them and they are everywhere. Whereas it is possible to avoid alcohol and other drugs, it is nigh-on impossible to avoid sugar and wheat on a daily basis.

Of course, you could go down this route and cut them out for ever. Some people do manage it and it works well for them, so if you can and want to, that's fine.

What we have seen over the years is that the vast majority of us don't manage to cut them out completely. In fact, trying to cut these foods out of our diets altogether makes us obsess about them even more, even if the reason for wanting to avoid them makes complete sense or has scientific validity. The deprivation fuels the *feeling* of addiction and when we give in, we eat and eat and eat and it feels like we cannot stop.

Is this just our biology? Is it just a physical response? It's just as likely that the deprivation plays as big a part in the craving as the substance itself. Even when we know incontrovertibly that it would be beneficial to us to avoid a particular food for a very good reason, this knowledge alone is not enough to stop us craving it. We might know and believe that it is not good for us in any way, and yet we obsess about it. And even when we do manage to remove it from our diet, do we stop overeating for ever or do we simply overeat something else instead? If we use food as a way to manage, cope, distract, treat, etc., not over-eating sugar or wheat or whatever may well mean that we turn to something else instead. Overeating is overeating whether it's carrot cake or carrot sticks.

BE YOUR OWN GURU

We encourage you to be your own guru. Experiment for your-self to find out if there are foods that you cannot stop eating – foods that feel like a drug to you. Make a list of these foods and then tune in when you eat them. Make a note of how you feel after you've eaten them, and whether eating them makes you want to eat more of these specific foods or more in general. You can then decide if you are overeating them because you are physiologically addicted or if you are overeating them for other reasons.

WHAT ABOUT FOODS WE *CAN'T* EAT?

Of course, if there are foods you can't or don't eat for ethi-cal, religious or medical reasons and you never overeat them, then that's fine, the tools in this chapter do not apply to you. What we are talking about here is when setting yourself rigid dietary restrictions or having lists of good and bad foods leads to craving and then overeating the very foods you want to avoid.

If, on the other hand, you have an intolerance or an allergy, or you have diabetes for example, but you still sometimes find yourself overeating the foods that make you feel ill, here's a thought. Often, because they make us ill we tell ourselves we *can't* have them. In fact, that's not really true. We *can* have them, in the sense that there's nothing stopping us putting them in our mouths, chewing and swallowing. We *can* eat them. So rather than telling ourselves we can't, it can be empowering and affirming to recognise that we are *choosing* not to because we know what the consequences will be. We are *choosing* to put our health and wellbeing before our taste buds. And, at the same time, we can tune in to our feelings and our thoughts (see pp. 115–7) and acknowledge how we feel about it – pissed off or sad, hard done by or whatever – and we'll be showing you how to deal with all of that in the coming chapter.

STOCKING UP

Once we have identified our forbidden foods (see Chapter 5), we can move on to the next step, stocking up.

Pick one of the foods on your forbidden-food list and go out and buy lots of it. More than you could possibly eat all in one go. You will need to stock up several times, to make sure that you always have more than you could eat. There is a good reason for this: scarcity creates demand – if you think it's running out, you are more likely to finish it all off. So make sure there's plenty: abundance is key. And as soon as levels go down, replenish. You have to believe that *whenever* you want this food, you will have it, then it will start to lose its magic power.

If it's not something you can easily stock up on, like delivery pizza or a creamy latte from your favourite coffee shop, then make sure you buy it whenever you want it. Make it a daily pit stop. Organise regular takeaways and home deliveries. Make sure you have it as often as you can and want to.

You won't have to stock up on *all* your forbidden foods in turn. You will have to go through several of them, and eventually your brain gets the message. You'll start to believe that you will let yourself have what you want and that nothing is forbidden. Start with one and take it from there.

Take the food out of its packaging

It's a good idea to take the food out of its packaging, wherever possible. Fill a gigantic Tupperware with crisps, unwrap your bars of chocolate, break them up and store the squares in a sealed container. When the food is not stored in pre-packed portions, you can choose just how much you want based on the size of your appetite and you won't be tempted to polish off what's left just because there are a few left in the pack. A spaghetti jar full of peanuts or Maltesers will suddenly make the idea of fun size, family size, grab bags and share bags irrelevant.

IT'S NOT A TREAT

This isn't a treat to have after you've eaten your greens. Have it as your starter, main and pudding. Make a meal of it, have it for breakfast, lunch and dinner. To truly legalise these foods, they need to be readily available and you need to have them whenever you want them. If they stay a treat, they stay special and if they stay special, they stay forbidden.

Sit down, put it on a plate and focus

When we eat in front of the TV it's so easy to munch our way through a pack or two of crisps without even noticing. Likewise, when we grab lunch and eat it at the computer, we barely register what we've eaten. It's so easy to eat and eat and eat with repeated trips to the fridge or on the go when doing a thousand other things. We miss the experience, we barely taste what we're eating and often end up eating more than we need. When we sit down, put the food on a plate and focus, we acknowledge to ourselves that we are eating – we make it official. When eating *is* the activity, we are much less likely to overeat. Have a go and see what a difference this can make. When you eat your forbidden foods, put them on a plate, sit down and eat them with awareness.

SO IS THIS GOODBYE TO CHOCOLATE?

So if you legalise chocolate, for example, which is definitely a number-one forbidden food, does that mean you'll never overeat it again?

Sometimes, the main reason we overeat chocolate is *because* it's forbidden. We tell ourselves we shouldn't have it, we try to resist and it's that very deprivation that fuels our desire – eventually, we give in and overeat it. The trigger in this situation *is* the deprivation. We don't want anything else, only chocolate will do. If there wasn't any chocolate, we wouldn't be overeating in that moment. By stocking up and legalising chocolate, we'll stop craving it. And, overeating is a complex business, so even when we've legalised it and we no longer overeat it *just* because it's chocolate, it may still be our food of choice when we over-eat for all those other reasons: because we're lonely, bored or pissed off or because we feel bad saying no . . . It's not specifically about the chocolate in these cases; if it wasn't chocolate, we'd still be overeating – just something else. And in those situations even though deprivation isn't part of the equation, we tend to choose our favourite food; chocolate. By legalising our forbidden foods, we eliminate all the overeating we do which is fuelled by deprivation alone and for some of us, that's a lot of chocolate!

With *Beyond Temptation*, you're learning to stop overeating whatever the reason and whatever the food, whether it's triggered by deprivation or not. In the next chapter you'll discover the tools to manage when the overeating is not about just the food.

WARNING!

If you think this is a recipe for disaster, and you're tempted to skip this step altogether – since you're going to learn how to stop overeating anyway – think again. Not legalising your forbidden foods will backfire. If a food stays forbidden, you will keep overeating it, however many tools you have at your disposal.

No forbidden foods?

If you really, truly don't have any forbidden foods, this chapter is not for you. Ignore it and focus on what we've been doing up to now.

TAKE ACTION

Stock up and legalise your forbidden foods. One at a time.

Step-by-step guide to stocking up

Step 1 Choose one item from your forbidden-food list.

Step 2 Go out and buy *loads* of it or make regular pit stops.

Step 3 Take the food out of its packaging.

Step 4 Eat when you want it.

Step 5 Keep replenishing stocks, so levels never get low.

YOUR **ACTION** CHECKLIST

☐ **Make it official**: call it overeating

☐ **Observe yourself with curiosity:** overeat with awareness

☐ **Identify your triggers**: find out why you overeat

☐ **Lighten the load:** talk about what it's really like

☐ **Find out about your forbidden foods:** make a list

→

☐ **Tune in to your Gremlin:** get to know it

☐ **Tune in to your feelings:** name and acknowledge them

☐ **Tune in to your overeating body:** listen to your body talk

☐ **Pause:** for just one minute

☐ **Stock up:** legalise your forbidden foods

•

CHAPTER ELEVEN

The Overeater's Secret Superpowers

YOU ARE ABOUT TO DISCOVER three tools that will change your life for ever. You can call on anyone of your secret superpowers at any time, anywhere, in any type of situation, whenever you feel the need to go beyond temptation.

Ok, they're not *really* superpowers, although, there is something very powerful and quite magical about them. Experiment with them and you will find that you are no longer at the mercy of your Gremlin or controlled by your emotions or paralysed by your overeating body. You will feel normal and in control around food. And that's super powerful.

SUPERPOWER 1 · THE 1-MINUTE MANTRA

Now that you know all about your Gremlin and how it talks you into overeating, we are going to introduce you to a way of dealing with it so that *you* are in charge, *you* make the decisions and *you* choose whether or not to overeat. We call it the 1-minute mantra.

When our Gremlins have the upper hand, we feel powerless, immobilised and defenceless in the face of what can sometimes feel like an unstoppable urge to eat. All the research you've been doing, all the information you have gathered, is powerful ammunition. The moment you notice your Gremlin and see it for what it is – as soon as you are aware – you are no longer at its mercy. Once you can recognise those unhelpful thoughts as your Gremlin, you can take charge and make different choices.

The most effective way to make sure that you are the boss and you call the shots is not to get caught up in the content of a Gremlin's rants, whines, pleas or attacks. Avoid all argument or discussion. If you've been taking action and tuning in, you'll know that your Gremlin will say just the thing to press your buttons or to pull at your heart strings. It's been doing it for such a long time. Entering into a discussion with it, trying to explain, reason, justify or win an argument is doomed to failure. It will always get the better of you and will always seek to have the last word.

Your Gremlin wants you to believe that what it says is the only truth – that you *are* your Gremlin. So the secret is not to engage with it, even for moment. Once you've caught it in action, step back and watch it. All you'll need is your 1-minute mantra.

Create your 1-minute mantra

Your 1-minute mantra is a word or phrase that you have pre-pared in advance and that you can repeat, broken-record style, for up to a minute, with force and determination, if necessary, until your Gremlin either backs down and you have shut it up or it has run out of steam. Your mantra is a simple phrase that you can remember easily and that your Gremlin will eventually stop arguing or pleading with. We use the word 'mantra' because, as you'll see, you will need to repeat it several times, mantra style.

The tone and intention with which you say your mantra are as important as the words you use. Of course, you won't necessarily be saying it out loud. You'll be saying it in your head, to your Gremlin. Only you will know whether your Gremlin needs to meet a firm, strong response, a humorous teasing tone, a reassuring, loving one or the verbal equivalent of a dismissive shrug. For particularly harsh, critical and angry Gremlins, you will need to muster a firm, decisive, no-argument tone. You may need to talk loudly or even shout. If your Gremlin is pathetic, weak and needy, you'll need to be the grown-up, the knowing adult, with a bit of compassion and kindness. At times, humour can really hit the spot; our Gremlins take themselves so seriously, and most of them don't have an ounce of humour, so making fun of them, patronising, ridiculing and shushing them up often works a treat.

The best way to create your own mantra is to start with your Gremlin's favourite catchphrases. If you've been journaling or making notes as you've worked through the previous chapters, look back over what you've written to help you identify what *your* Gremlin's catchphrases are: how does it talk you into overeating? What does it say to goad, bully, reassure or seduce you, so that you end up with you hand in the biscuit tin?

Once you know what tactics your Gremlin uses and what its favourite catchphrases are, have a go at coming up with a short, sweet mantra that clearly and firmly shows that you won't be bulldozed and you won't give in. Make it short and snappy. And remember, no explanations, justifications or stories.

Here are some mantras we know work:

Be quiet

Shut up

Enough

Fuck off

Piss off

Whatever

Yeah, and?

Blablabla

Shhhhhh . . .

Mmmm . . .

STOP

That's not helpful

Shoo

Shush

That's enough

You're not welcome

There, there

Ah, I know . . .

Practice makes perfect

Don't wait until the moment you are overeating to try and think of a mantra. That's when you are at your most vulnerable, so you need to be prepared. Have a look at the list of mantras above now. Do you have a sense of which one will work for you and the tone you will say it with?

Whatever you mantra, your Gremlin will try everything to make you engage with it and it will try to engage with you. It knows that the way to get you to overeat is by getting you caught up in a dialogue. The idea is to cut off the dialogue. Stick with your mantra.

If it helps, you can visualise an imaginary barrier between you and your Gremlin. Conjure this image when you use your mantra. It could be a perspex wall, an iron curtain, a force field, a shutter, a brick wall.

After a bit of practice, you may find that your mantra needs tweaking or a slightly different tone or you might have to change it and experiment with a different one. You'll only find out by using it and seeing what happens.

This isn't goodbye

Our Gremlins do not vanish or disappear for ever. However determined and persistent we are, they will always be there in one form or another. For as long as you can think, you will have Gremlins. The aim is not to get rid of them, but to be aware of them. Awareness gives us choice and choice gives us freedom. By getting to know how your overeating Gremlin operates, by being so tuned in to it that you catch it the minute it starts, you'll be able to silence it quickly and without a fight. Eventually, it will go quiet.

Some Gremlins then morph and try a different tack to get you back to your old behaviours; their existence depends on you staying the same and overeating, so their agenda is to make sure you stay stuck in old, familiar patterns. And the more you shine a light on them, bringing them into your awareness and taking charge, the less power they have, so that eventually, when you hear your Gremlin at work, you find yourself smiling at it.

SUPERPOWER 2 · THE FEELINGS TOOL-KIT

As we saw in Chapter 5, the first step in dealing with our feelings is being able to recognise, name and acknowledge them. If we don't know what we are feeling, there's not much we can do about it. And once you can name your feelings, you're ready to use the feelings tool-kit.

The feelings tool-kit is a set of four straightforward strategies to help you manage your feelings. They are tools to help you connect with your anger, fear, sadness and happiness and stay in control. They are tools that you can experiment with and then make your own.

At the end of the day, the *only* way to stop eating our feelings away is to be willing to acknowledge and deal with whatever we would feel if we were not eating. There are no two ways about it. We can distract ourselves as much as we like, unless we are willing to dip our toe into the discomfort of unfamiliar and un-comfortable feelings, we will eventually come back to the food.

Feel it

Feel the feeling, rather than eating it away. As you may have already discovered, sometimes just allowing ourselves to *name* a feeling, to recognise it and acknowledge it, without resisting, fighting or having judgments about it, is enough to dissipate it.

When we say *feel it*, we are not suggesting that it is ok to dump your feelings on someone else, to moan, to rant or to lash out at them. This is for your benefit only. Feeling your feelings is about finding a safe way to feel sad and cry, feel angry and rant, feel afraid and shake, feel elated and express your happiness.

Feeling your feelings does not mean *thinking* about your feelings or analysing them. It doesn't mean that you go over and over the situation or event that triggered the feeling in your mind. It means focusing on *feeling*. Feel it with your body, let the emotion flow through you.

Sometimes we talk ourselves out of our feelings by telling ourselves it really doesn't matter. Someone might say something that hurts us and we tell ourselves they didn't mean it. We feel angry and we tell ourselves there's no point, we can't change the situation anyway or maybe we think we deserved what we got. We judge our feelings as silly or tell ourselves we are overreacting. Feeling our feelings is about allowing them to surface without having to be reasonable or justified or right. Feeling our feelings is simply about becoming aware of what's there, what's bubbling up inside us and allowing it to come up, no matter what.

It doesn't matter that your mother didn't mean to upset you when commenting on your weight. If you feel upset by it, you feel upset. The fact that your boss was right, that you *had* made a mistake, doesn't make your anger any less valid. If you feel angry with him, that's all that matters. It makes no difference whether you think it's irrational or silly or selfish or pointless or ugly or out of proportion to feel desperate because your boyfriend has just called to say he can't make tonight. You feel desperate – and criticising yourself for it won't make it go away.

You don't have to have a good reason for feeling the way you do. You don't have to be able to make it right or *be* right, get revenge or make someone feel sorry or see sense. Your feelings don't have to be justified, nor do they have to be reasonable or proportionate. The aim here is to get your feelings out of your system, so that you don't eat to stuff them down or avoid them. And whether they are justified or make sense to you or not, you're feeling them anyway – so stuffing your feelings down with food, reasoning yourself out of them or pretending they are not there doesn't work in the long term. In fact, stuffing our feelings down or pushing them away, keeping a lid on them or eating to deal with them is exhausting and can, ultimately, lead to depression and illness.

What would it be like to curl up on your bed and sob your heart out, instead of numbing away the pain with a cup of tea and a packet of biscuits?

Can you imagine stamping your feet, beating your fists and hurling obscenities and insults at an imaginary wrongdoer, having a good old tantrum, rather than munching furiously on one crisp after another? What it is *like* to feel anxious, to fidget, to shake, to sweat, when you don't push the fear away and stuff it down with another helping of mashed potato? How would it be to skip and jump and scream and let yourself be giddy with joy or excitement, instead of celebrating with another scoop of ice cream?

Feelings don't last for ever

All feelings will come to an end. Just like the packet of biscuits, the bag of crisps, the bowl of mashed potato, the tub of ice cream – you will get to the bottom of your feelings, they *will* end. They will not go on for ever. In fact, when you allow yourself to feel your feelings and stop fighting or resisting them, you may well find that they come and go quite quickly.

You don't have to feel and wallow in your feelings for ages. To start with, one way to ensure that you don't get lost in your feelings is to set a time limit. So when you want to use this tool – when you are going to allow yourself to feel your feelings – decide how long you want to do it for. Start small, maybe just a couple of minutes. Then set a timer and when the time is up, stop, decide if you want more time and repeat, if necessary. Keep going until you've had enough.

If the feeling persists and there seems to be no end in sight, if it goes on and on and on, remember that you have a whole host of other tools you can draw on in this chapter. Remember also that the way you think impacts the way you feel, so it could be helpful to go back to your mantra and make sure your Gremlin is not at work. You might be fuelling the feelings by thinking about and analysing the situation. Remember, the key here is not to *think* about the feeling: just *feel* it. And, as you'll see in later on in this chapter, working with your overeating body can help you manage your feelings too.

Explore it

Putting your feelings into words or drawing a picture can be helpful in making sense of what can sometimes feel like an impenetrable tangle of thoughts and emotions.

Pouring it all out in a journal, giving your feelings colours and shapes on paper, writing a letter to someone (that you will never send) where you can vent, reflect or question what you're feeling, instead of shutting yourself off and turning to food, can provide helpful insights and even closure. And, as you are doing this, remember to focus on feeling, rather than thinking. Thinking about it is likely to keep you stuck; feeling whatever it is, as you explore, will help the emotions to rise and fall, to come and then go.

Share it

Share it with people who understand what you're doing and won't judge you or try to make it better. It could be a good friend, a therapist or a member of your family. In our experience, people who don't know what the Beyond Temptation approach is about might find it difficult to support you in a way that's helpful. If they are not comfortable with *their* feelings, they are unlikely to be comfortable with yours.

Sometimes our feelings are big and frightening and sharing them with someone who cares or with someone who has the professional skills to offer guidance and support is the wisest thing to do.

One of the best places we know to share them is on the Beyond Chocolate Forum. It's open 24/7 and there are dozens of threads which you can post on or just read for reassurance. One in particular is called 'I need support'. The forum is a hugely caring and welcoming environment and can make all the difference. There's something valuable about knowing that you're not on your own – that hundreds of women have experienced something close to what you're going through, and understand and speak the same language. (For information about joining the forum see Log On for More, p. 245.)

Contain it

If it's not the right place or the right time to feel your feelings or explore them or share them, or if they just feel too big and you need more support, one way to manage your feelings is to contain them, in an imaginary safe box.

The first step is to tune in and become aware of what it is you're feeling. Name it. Acknowledge how you are feeling and then imagine putting that feeling in a virtual safe box.

This is not about ignoring your feelings or pushing them away; the point of using an imaginary safe box is to store them temporarily, until you are in a place and at a time that feels safe and appropriate to take them out and engage with them. So when you decide to contain your feelings by putting them in your box, make sure you set a time and a place when you will open the box up again and take them out. This will mean waiting until you are alone or in another place or until you have the right type of support to help you with it. When you are ready, use one of the other tools from the feelings tool-kit; feel it, explore it or share it.

Create your safe box

What does *your* safe box look like? Imagine it. How big is it? What materials is it made of? What colour is it? How does it lock? Create a crystal-clear picture in your mind so that when your feelings surface and it's not a good time, you know exactly where to put them. You might even draw a picture of your safe box to make it more real.

So when your mum makes a comment about how much weight you've put on or your boss bollocks you or your boyfriend calls to cancel and you're in the middle of the supermarket, clock the feeling, name it, imagine yourself putting it in the box and closing it. Then take a deep breath and decide when you'll open it up.

Whatever you do, don't let the feelings fester away in your box. Commit yourself to opening it up, take yourself gently by the hand and *do* it. There's no feeling too big or too small to fit into your box. Adjust the size of your box to match the size of your feeling. However, there's only room for *one* feeling at a time in there. You can't keep putting feelings in and leaving them. You have to take one out before you put another one in.

And if, when you go back to open the box, it feels as if the feeling has gone away, that you don't feel it any more, give yourself a few minutes to recall the incident or the situation. Take yourself back there. A feeling doesn't just disappear, though naming it and acknowledging it *can* sometimes be all you need. Just make sure you are not pretending it's all ok before you put your box away. Give yourself some time to feel or explore or share it and see what comes up.

SUPERPOWER 3 • BODY TALK

As we saw in Chapter 6, we all have an overeating body. We embody our thoughts, our feelings and our urge to overeat. Whatever we are feeling, thinking and doing, our bodies tell the story.

When you tune in and recognise what you are doing with your body, how you are forming and shaping your experience or how your overeating body is impacting the way you feel, you can choose to reorganise your body and that, in turn, will have an impact on your experience. Reorganising your body simply means tuning in and changing what you are doing with the various parts of your body, with awareness.

When you disorganise anxiety or anger or, indeed, any feeling, when you disorganise the body that shapes your feelings, you lessen their intensity and the feelings become more manageable. This is indeed a superpower: having the skill to regulate your feelings in this way works so much better than doing it with food.

Reorganising body talk

Tune in to your overeating body (see Chapter 6 for a step-by-step guide).

Start with your breathing. Entire philosophies are centred around the breath, so we won't go into the whys and wherefores here. Suffice to say that changing your breathing can change your whole experience. Taking deep, steady breaths, allowing oxygen to flow into your system and breathing out fully works miracles.

Once you have noticed *how* you are breathing, you can experiment with breathing more deeply or more slowly or more steadily, whatever helps.

Next, reorganise your **posture**. If you are slumped, experiment with straightening your spine – ground yourself by placing both feet on the floor. Do it slowly, gradually. If you are rigid, start moving, stretch, maybe stand up or walk, give your body a shake.

Next, reorganise your different **body parts**: your feet, legs, thighs, buttocks, hips, abdomen, chest, arms, hands, shoulders, back, neck. If you are tense and tight, experiment with softening each muscle. Do the same with the muscles in your **face**: your mouth, eyes, jaw, cheeks, lips, teeth, etc.

Notice how reorganising your body talk is impacting any internal sensations. If your heart is still beating very fast, or you are aware of a constricting feeling in your chest or pain anywhere (or any pain, discomfort), you may need to spend more time tuning in and reorganising your body talk. Take it slowly, gradually, one step at a time.

How do you feel in your clothes? Loosen anything that's tight, take something off, if you're hot.

Whatever you are closing, experiment with opening up. Whatever you are stiffening or tightening, experiment with softening and releasing. Whatever is collapsing and heavy, give it some form by straightening or firming.

You get the picture? The way you hold your body will impact how you feel. Try to imagine feeling furious while breathing deeply and slowly, relaxing all the muscles in your face and your body and sitting softly in your chair. Have a go, do it now.

Whatever you become aware of when you tune in, experiment with reorganising your body talk. Lessen or increase the intensity. Whether you are softening or making yourself more solid, reorganising your body talk will change your experience.

TAKE ACTION

The next time you overeat, pick one of your superpowers to experiment with:

- Practise your 1-minute mantra.

- Explore, feel, contain or share whatever you're feeling.

- Reorganise your body talk.

YOUR **ACTION** CHECKLIST

☐ **Make it official**: call it overeating

☐ **Observe yourself with curiosity:** overeat with awareness

☐ **Identify your triggers**: find out why you overeat

☐ **Lighten the load:** talk about what it's really like

☐ **Find out about your forbidden foods:** make a list

→

☐ **Tune in to your Gremlin:** get to know it

☐ **Tune in to your feelings**: name and acknowledge them

☐ **Tune in to your overeating body:** listen to your body talk

☐ **Pause:** for just one minute

☐ **Stock up:** legalise your forbidden foods

☐ **Experiment with your superpowers:** 1-minute mantra, feelings tool-kit, body talk

CHAPTER TWELVE

•

Women in Action

WHAT IS IT LIKE TO EXPERIMENT with pausing? What is it like to tune in? What happens when we legalise our forbidden foods? They are very different experiences for each one of us. There's no right or wrong way to use your 1-minute mantra. There's nothing that you're *supposed to* realise when you experiment with the feelings tool-kit. There's nothing that you should be thinking or feeling when you reorganise your body talk. Whatever it's like for you, it's just fine. As long as you are taking action, however little, you'll be discovering something and that discovery is how you change.

Change is often a slow process – small steps, little by little. In fact, it's generally better and longer lasting when it's slow, so finding a way to keep yourself motivated and to support your-self along the way can make all the difference. Keeping a journal, posting on the forum, writing a blog, talking about it, making charts or drawing spider diagrams, sharing it with like-minded people, documenting your experience in some way – all of this is very helpful and gives you an opportunity to reflect on what you're discovering, to acknowledge and log the process as you experiment. It's so encouraging to look back after a few months and see just how far you've come.

SO MANY WOMEN ... EXPERIMENTING ...

Our friends are not quite ready to stop yet, they will be very soon. They just need a bit more time to practise using everything they've learned so far. Let's see how they're getting on.

Alice (private diary entry on her laptop)

Dear Diary,

I've done it. I never thought I would. I was halfway through a croissant and I put it down. I'm shaking. Deep breath. It's ok. I'm ok. I used my mantra, I told little miss goody-goody to be quiet and she stopped.

I give myself such a hard time. Sometimes, I think the only time I let myself relax a bit is when I eat something nice. I try so hard to be good, to get it right. I am a perfectionist, aren't I? I always thought that was a good thing. But if it's not, then I'm not sure what to do.

What am I so scared of? I don't know, but I'm scared. I'm scared of putting on weight, I'm scared of messing up, I'm scared that everyone will see that I'm not as in control as they think I am. So is this it then? Maybe what I need to do is feel the fear. That's what they said in the book. Feel it.

Well I'm feeling it and it's ok for the moment. It's not as bad as I thought it would be. Maybe I'm not doing it right. My Gremlin keeps telling me I have to get it right. I have to work hard, I have to. And I have to be careful, I have to watch what I eat. I can't put on weight. I really can't. Oh, there she goes again. Be quiet, little miss goody-goody. It's such hard work, it's so stressful being me sometimes. Be quiet. I know I'm not really that overweight, but compared to Karen and Catherine I am. How do they do it? How do they stay that thin? I know it's up to me. I know I can't keep on eating like this and going to the gym every day. There's got to be another way, there must be. I just don't know what it is yet.

Alice x

Becky (handwritten stream of consciousness)

Monday 23 June. I couldn't pause. I really wanted to pause, but I just couldn't. It felt like I'd physically explode if I didn't eat. I was standing at the buffet and I felt so sick and full up. My belly was straining against my waistband and I knew I didn't need any more, but this little whiney voice inside my head (I suppose that's my Gremlin) kept pleading and begging. I just went blank. I think I was so tense and scared I just went on automatic pilot. I know this doesn't mean I've failed. It was just a pause. It's ok to eat, anyway. If anyone was reading this, they'd think I was mad. I don't know what to do next. What if I can't ever stop? What if I'm one of those people who just eat and eat and can never stop? What if I just keep getting fatter? I know this isn't helpful. I know. It's not helpful. It's not helpful. I'm going to tune in. I'm going to do it now. I can do that and maybe it will help. Feelings, how am I feeling? Scared. I'm scared. Thoughts. What's my Gremlin saying? Well it was saying all those things about me never being able to change and getting fatter. And right now? Er . . . seems to have gone quiet. Body talk? I'm tensing my thighs and bum. God this is hard.

Christine (a page in her black Moleskine notebook)

Wednesday 16 January. I've put the jelly beans in a jar. It's massive. Lucy thought it was for the patients at first and thought I'd gone mad, so I had to put it in my room instead. Every time I walk past them my heart skips a beat. I keep on turning round to check if anyone is watching before I realise they're in full view and it's not a secret any more. I keep rummaging in my pockets for them and being surprised they're empty. It's so automatic that I don't realise I've done it until I do. I think my

Gremlin hasn't caught on yet. Or I'm not hearing it, anyway. There's no dialogue or anything like that. It's only when I come up empty-handed that I realise the Gremlin was at work. But I don't actually want them. I've hardly had any since I got the jar. I had lunch today. I actually went to the café with Lucy and Ben and had a salad. It was really nice to sit and chat and eat. I think this might work.

Debbie (forum post)

> Debs16
> Thread: I want to celebrate
> Topic: Great Week!

I'M SO HAPPY!!!

I have been stocking up and tuning in this week. It's incredible I've been eating what I want, enjoying it and I'm not overeating half as much! I've been taking my time food shopping and going around and looking at foods I wouldn't usually buy and getting ideas for meals, as I wanted to plan and be organised, as I knew I had a busy week. I also made a concerted effort to cook every night, even though it was just for me as my hubby is working away. And because I have had exactly what I wanted, I have not felt deprived once. I made sausage and mash one night and actually used real butter and 'proper' sausages and loved every mouthful. And you know, when I actually looked at my plate of food I was actually eating LESS than if I has been doing it the Slimming World way, but I was eating better-quality, more satisfying food. So satisfying, in fact, I didn't want any dessert until about two hours later (unheard of for me!). I have also swapped horrible 'light' yoghurts for Longley Farm live yoghurts (no additives) which I adored as a kid and are also SOOO satisfying.

I also decided to jot everything down that I ate – not in an obsessive 'diet diary' way, but so that I could keep an idea of meals for future reference. I feel like a light bulb has finally clicked on.

Replies:

That's great news. Good to hear you are doing so well.

Congratulations, very inspiring! xx

Lovely to hear your progress this week Debs – fantastic!!!

Good for you Debs. I have gone ten days and counting without having a binge. It may not seem like long but, apart from when I am on holiday (for some reason I eat less on holiday and usually lose weight), I haven't gone that long in six years. I have been feeding myself lots of yummy foods and making sure I am satisfied and full. I have changed my exercise regime and am learning to like my body more. Here's to another ten days.

Emily (online journal entry)

I've had it. I can't do this any more. I won't. I fucking won't.
I refuse to live a double life, what for the rest of my days?
Am I supposed to do this for ever? I just don't think I can.
Enough, I have had enough.

I tuned in a few minutes ago and all I could think of was
how angry I was. And I've decided, I'm going to tell him
and if he doesn't like it, if he doesn't like me, if he stops
loving me . . . Oh Christ, I don't know what I'll do, but it
can't be worse than how I'm feeling now. It just can't be.
I have the right to eat what I want. He may not agree,
but I don't want to pretend any more. I do it so much –
pretending. I pretend that I agree with Emma when she says
that children need a set bedtime, I pretend I don't mind
when Sandra doesn't come to my parties, I pretend that I
don't mind when Adam forgets to wish me a happy birthday.
I'm going to stop pretending. I'll start with being a veggie
and I'll take it from there. Talk about diving right into the
deep end. God, this feels good. Really good. And terrifying.
And exciting.

Fatima (blog post)

www.hungrygirl.com

News flash! A friend has warned me that my father knows
about this blog. So dear readers, if everything suddenly
goes quiet, you'll know my cover's blown. Keep your fingers
crossed. My life won't be worth living if he has found out.

Anyway, moving swiftly on and getting to the point of this post while I still can. I've been experimenting with tuning in and getting to know my Gremlin and it's not been uneventful. On Monday night, after everyone had gone to sleep, I was up in my room revising (as usual) and I suddenly got it. I realised I was feeling furious. Initially, I thought it was sadness, which may sound a bit odd, but bear with me. I tuned in and I just kept coming up with 'I'm feeling unhappy'. So I asked myself, 'Unhappy about what?' and the answer was, 'unhappy with the fact that Daddy (stop sniggering, I know I'm too old to call him that) thinks he can tell me what to eat'. So anyway, you know how some people say, 'I'm very unhappy with this . . .' but they don't sound unhappy, they sound cross, well I realised that I was cross. I'm so cross with him I could scream. Scary and liberating all wrapped into one. I have no idea what I'm going to do with this information just yet, but I know there's something in it.

So then I thought I'd see if I could tune in to what I was thinking. And this is the really odd bit, my Gremlin has mutated. She used to be all terrified and pathetic, but now she was ranting and raving and being really rather bold. When I tuned in to my thoughts, I realised I was sort of having an imaginary conversation with my father. I'm going to try to reproduce it here, more for my benefit than yours. It was definitely a monologue and it went something like this: Why can't you see that I'm old enough to decide for myself what I eat? I don't need to you tell me what I can and can't have. I don't need your diet plans and I really hate it when you weigh me. I really, really hate it.

And the body talk was telling too. I was tapping my foot and kind of hammering my fists on the table.

So what do I do with these thoughts and feelings? I can't tell him any of it. He'd have a fit and I'd never hear the end of it. And it wouldn't make any difference, anyway. He wouldn't take any notice. He's not going to stop just because I tell him to. Something's got to change though because I can't keep going on like this.

Til next time . . . (let's hope there is one).

Grace (video diary)

Hello. Well here I am again. Fucking hell, Saturday night and instead of being out with Megan having fun, I'm sitting here doing all this soul searching. She called earlier and said she has to work late again. It hurts. So much. I feel so sad, I could drown in it, I feel so sad. I can hear that fucker in my head going on about how crap I am, how I deserve this, how she doesn't love me. I so want to eat. There is a tightness in my chest, it feels like my heart is breaking. My throat is so tight that it hurts to swallow. My temples are buzzing and it feels like my eyeballs are on fire. It's like I'm burning, everywhere. I know, I know now that I do this to myself. Megan is staying away because she can't bear to watch me erase myself any more. I know that I have to stop hiding behind her, stop letting her live for me . . . stop sitting at home eating and watching telly. Fuck I want that ice cream. No! No I don't.

Ice cream is not the answer. What I want is to start living.
To stop hiding. I want to get excited about something other
than fucking ice cream. I think I can. I know I can. I'm going to
call Megan, I'm going to tell her I love her. Over and out.

Heather (recorded on her mobile-phone voice memo)

I'm sitting here in the McDonald's car park. My voice is
so shaky. I'm shaky all over. I've set the timer and I've
promised myself I'll go in and order when it goes off. I
don't know what to do. I can't breathe. I feel sick. I keep
on thinking of the chips, of the hot, crunchy chips. I'm
fat. This is who I am. I'm fatty, chubs, the fat one. I eat
burgers because I don't know how to be anybody else.
Who would I be if I wasn't fat? My heart is pounding.
Beeeeep. That's the timer. I don't want to get out of the
car and walk in there. If I stop eating burgers, I can be
someone else. I don't know if I can do that. I don't know
if I can not be me. But I want to stop overeating. It's
killing me, I hate it. Oh God, I just don't know. I've been
thinking about this constantly, it's all I can think about.

Who am I? I am a woman; I am a confused woman; I
am a good listener; I am a film lover; I am a reader of good
books; I am a loyal friend; I know how to organise things.

I'm going to stop now, exhausted. Going to drive home
and have a bath.

Isabelle (journal)

I sit here in my kitchen in the dark and smoke
cigarettes and feel sorry for myself, greasy tears
running down my cheeks. It doesn't feel good. I
pooh-pooh the little child howling for her mother
and remind myself that I am an adult now. I'm torn
between anger and self-pity. Anger at him and at
myself and at my good old friend self-pity. That safe,
warm cocoon of desperation and longing that I know
so well and that beckons me like a chocolate cake,
like a warm, syrupy tart, like a thousand gummy
sugar bears. I will myself to feel the anger, really
feel it and I tell the self-pity to piss off. How could
he show up at my party, MY PARTY, the culmination
of eighteen years, my shining golden moment, with
his pathetic happiness, with his oh-so-perfect
little girlfriend whose shiny brown hair and good
manners mock my tomboy looks, my spotty chin and
my dumpy bulges. The little girl inside me rebels at
the thought: she tears her hair out and stamps her
feet and screams and bellows in rage. The little
girl who was only loved conditionally, cannot bear
not be loved. And I am tormented: what does she

have that I do not? How is she better? Why does she deserve him more than me? Why am I not good enough?

I will go to bed now, heavy hearted and still angry. I thought that I had digested the pain, but it sits there in my stomach like a brick, heavy and solid. And no matter how much I vomit, I cannot get rid of it. It has settled deep down inside me and causes me constant discomfort. I am hoping that this royal rant will serve to strengthen me, that it will help to crumble the brick inside my stomach into fine dust that I can shit away tomorrow instead of throwing it up. At least I haven't eaten and that feels good. Rant over.

A day in the life of Jane

(fly-on-the-wall documentary script)

7.15 a.m. – kitchen

A baby sits in a high chair, banging his spoon and sending flecks of soggy cereal flying around the room. He has Weetabix smeared all over his face and in his hair. Next to him, a toddler is sitting at the table wailing hysterically, 'Not the red one! I don't want the red one, Mummy! I want the orange one!'

Jane is battling with the door of the dishwasher which is stuck and won't open, while trying to push the cat out of the way with her foot. She grabs the offending piece of toast from her daughter and starts eating it while she makes another one – this time with orange marmalade. She looks at the mess surrounding her and thinks, *How am I supposed to stop and PAUSE for goodness sake? Look at me, I haven't got the time to wee!*

10 a.m. – kitchen

Jane is sifting through a load of laundry and occasionally walks over to the hob to stir a stew which is bubbling away. Every time she does so, she has a little taste. Her little girl is sitting at the table scribbling all over the pages of a pretty pink journal with crayons, a half finished pot of yoghurt next to her. Jane looks at the child and thinks, *I bought that journal for me. I was going to use it to do the exercises from the book.* This is hopeless. She picks up the yoghurt pot and quickly eats what's left before throwing it away. We can hear the baby start crying. He's woken up.

12 p.m. – supermarket

Jane is walking up and down the aisles of the supermarket trying to blank out the insistent demands from her toddler, who wants everything, while keeping the little one from falling out of the trolley and breaking his neck. She grabs things off shelves without much thought, trying to get the ordeal over and done with as quickly as possible. She stops

in the bakery aisle and looks longingly at all the goodies
on display. She pauses to battle with herself: Ooooh I love
Cadbury's mini rolls. I shouldn't really, but I'm so tired. I
haven't had anything nice today. I can have one with a cuppa
when the kids are napping. Just one. Yeah right, I'll probably
end up eating the whole packet. It's just like it says in the
book. Once I start, I can't stop. It's true, I *do* use food as a treat.
It *does* help me to cope. I could use nap time to do some of
the exercises from the Gremlin chapter. I quite like the idea
of drawing mine. Yeah, but Sophia's drawn all over it. Maybe
tomorrow. Yes, tomorrow I'll go and buy a new one and then
I'll do it. I'm allowed a mini roll with my cup of tea. It's fine.
I'll make sure I just eat one.

2.30 p.m. – kitchen

Jane is alone in her kitchen. The house is quiet. She is standing
up at the counter drinking tea and eating one mini roll after
the other. Quickly, not thinking.

5 p.m. – kitchen

Jane is on the phone to her mother. They are having an
animated conversation. The phone is wedged between her
shoulder and her ear. She's cutting some fish fingers up at
the same time. She eats a few pieces quickly with her
fingers as she shares them out on to plates. At one point,
she freezes with her hand suspended in mid-air. 'Listen
Mum, I've got to go, I'll call you back later. Bye.' She puts the
phone down and looks at the chunk of fish finger in her

hand. *My God, I do this all the time! I've never realised how much I eat. I suppose I never thought of this as overeating. But it is. It really is. Gosh!* Her thoughts are interrupted by the baby who knocks over his cup of juice and she hurries off to clean up the mess.

7.45 p.m. – living room

The house is quiet. Jane is sitting on the sofa. A large glass of white wine and a bowl of peanuts are in front of her on the coffee table. She stares at them. Ok, what if I do the tuning in thing. I can. The kids are asleep – finally! – and Pete won't be home for at least another half hour. Dinner's ready. The laundry's done. I've still got to go through the baby's old clothes for the charity shop. Well, I can do that tomorrow. There's no rush. I could watch the new Great British Bake Off episode on iPlayer. I missed it last night. I wonder if the young guy is still in? They were doing bread. I love bread. No. Look at me, avoiding it. This is what I do, isn't it? I avoid everything. I could just sit here and watch it, drinking and eating peanuts. I'm so tired. I never have time like this. Ok, I'll have a go at tuning in and then switch the telly on.

7.48 p.m. – living room

Jane is sitting on the sofa. 'Umm, what's the first one? Oh yes, feelings. What am I feeling? Uhhhh, ummmm a bit panicky, actually. Yes, panicky. Ok, now Gremlin. What am I thinking? Well, I'm thinking about the wine and the peanuts. I'm thinking how much I want that first sip of wine. How lovely and salty the peanuts will be. I'm thinking how tired I am, how awful it's been today, how guilty I feel because I shouted at Tommy. What a bad mother I am. Actually, I'm not feeling panicky, I'm feeling despair. Can you change the feeling? Is that ok? I don't know. I don't know anything any more. Oh God, it's so complicated. I'm so tired. There I go again. Ok, how about my body? Everything aches, everything. My back is killing me from carrying the baby all day. My mouth is dry. I want to sleep! Oh! I want to sleep! Maybe I'll just put my feet up for a few minutes and close my eyes. Just until Pete gets home. Jane takes her shoes off and lies down on the sofa. She closes her eyes. The wine and the peanuts are on the table, untouched. The house is silent.

Kate (Excel spreadsheet)

Weekly tuning in log

MONDAY				
Overeating trigger	**Feeling**	**Thoughts**	**Body**	**Comment**
Thinking about this log.	Dread	Eat it and get rid of it. You know sugar is addictive. You won't rest until it's gone. Eat it and be done with it.	Eyes wide open and dry. Biting inside of cheek. Tense all over.	I so want to get this right. I ate the entire pack, so it wouldn't be in my way.

→

TUESDAY

Overeating trigger	Feeling	Thoughts	Body	Comment
Reading Stargazer's forum post about being wheat free for three months and then pigging out on cake at her best friend's hen do.	Agitated	Pff! Look, everyone does it. Don't be so wet. That rice milk is disgusting, anyway. Make the rice pudding with real milk. It's skimmed. It's fine.	Tense neck and shoulders Biting inside of cheek. Nostrils flared Knot in stomach.	Can't believe I fell for this! Ate the whole lot. Bloated, felt sick and had diarrhoea all night. Note: NO COW'S MILK – whatever the reason.

WEDNESDAY

Overeating trigger	Feeling	Thoughts	Body	Comment
Meeting Sally for tea at the Tea Rooms.	Panic	Oh stop effing about and make a decision! She's waiting. Just have the blimmin' toast. Thinly cut. Come on, stop faffing. It's not going to kill you just this once.	Staring down at menu without seeing it – everything blurred. Heart beating fast. Biting inside of cheek.	Stopped for croissant on the way home. Had three. The biting-cheek thing is obviously a clue. Note: watch out for cheek biting, it indicates overeating about to happen.

→

THURSDAY				
Overeating trigger	**Feeling**	**Thoughts**	**Body**	**Comment**
Lunch with Mum.	Furious	She does it on purpose. To taunt you. Go on, eat the crumble and get out of here. She's such a bitch.	Twiddling spoon. Muscles clenching. Lips pinched tight.	Love Mum's crumble, had two bowls. Couldn't resist.
				Interesting, when I'm angry I don't bite my cheek. But it's still about the mouth.
				Note: STOP going to Mum's for lunch.

FRIDAY				
Overeating trigger	**Feeling**	**Thoughts**	**Body**	**Comment**
NONE!!!!!	n/a	n/a	n/a	This is a first – result!

SATURDAY				
Overeating trigger	**Feeling**	**Thoughts**	**Body**	**Comment**
Not sure.	Not sure – stressed in general.	Don't know, was done eating before I realised.	Don't know, but inside of cheek is bleeding a little, so was probably at it again.	Not sure what happened today . . . feeling too confident from yesterday? Let my guard down?
				Note: be on the lookout.

→

SUNDAY				
Overeating trigger	**Feeling**	**Thoughts**	**Body**	**Comment**
Not sure (again).	Stressed	I don't know why you insist on eating that bloody quinoa – it is truly disgusting. There's some pasta left over from Harry's lunch. Do yourself a favour and finish it off.	Grinding teeth a little. Goosebumps Fists clenching.	Had all the pasta. I think the trigger may be the quinoa, but I'm not sure. Knew I wanted the pasta before I made the quinoa, so probably just an excuse. Feel fine having had the pasta. Note: experiment with eating pasta again and see what happens.

Leila (handwritten letter)

Dear Body

I've been working on my overeating for the past few weeks and I think it's going quite well. I'm not grazing so much during the day. Yesterday I didn't go to the kitchen once all afternoon. I wasn't trying not to, though. At one point, I noticed myself thinking about the chocolate biscuits in the cupboard, so I paused for a few seconds, told myself I could have them, if I really wanted them, then promptly forgot about them. That's amazing. What's wonderful about all this is that I've lost 2lb. I might even be able to get into those white jeans I used to love so much, if it carries on like this. I remember wearing them in Greece that summer — it must have been 2000 or 2001. I love that photo of James and me at the taverna. Those were the days . . .

I wanted to write this letter because it feels important to tell you that I'm doing everything

I can to change the things I don't like about you. I've started going to the gym again, so that should help and I've been religious about exfoliating and moisturising. I'm feeling really hopeful and positive for the first time in ages. I'm really looking forward to us being friends again. It's been such a long time. I'm sorry I've ignored you for so long.

Leila

Leila puts her pen in the other hand and lets her body write back . . .

Dear Leila

Thank you for writing to me. I'm glad we're back in contact. It does feel like you've been ignoring me for a long time. There's something I want to say to you and I hope you'll take it how it's meant — with love and good intention.

Leila, it doesn't matter how many pounds

you take off me or how much you exfoliate and tone me up, you can't lose the years. You can't go back in time. That holiday in Greece <u>was</u> lovely, but even if you do manage to get me back into those jeans, I'll look completely different. You and me, we're peri-menopausal, my skin is thinning and I think I've even noticed some age spots appearing on my hands. Stop fighting me, Leila. We're beautiful. We don't have to be frightened of getting older. Let's do it gracefully. Buy me some new jeans. Some that fit me and suit the shape I am now. I'd really like that.

I love you.

Your body

Natasha (spider diagram)

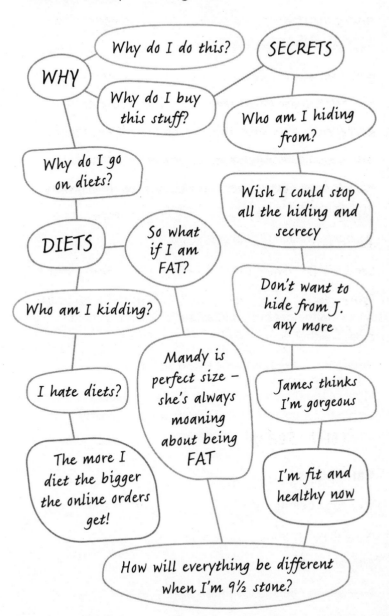

Olivia (computer log)

Friday 4 September

My Gremlin caricature

It's a thing, definitely a thing.

Old, very old. It's been there since the beginning of time.

It's a formless black goo. Like a cross between a golem and a sinister Mister Men character.

It's black. Its skin is cold and sticky.

It's quiet. It hisses at me and sometimes it shouts. But it's cold, always very cold.

It lurks in the deepest, darkest recesses of my mind, hiding, slithering around.

Where does it come from? Being adopted.

Most of the time it doesn't talk, just permeates everything with a thick, gelatinous coating of what I can only describe as a sense of inadequacy.

Catchphrases:

You don't belong.

No one wants you.

Why aren't I good enough?

Why doesn't he/she love me?

This is very helpful. I've never thought about it in these terms. I knew that being adopted was an issue, but I'd never seen it so clearly, especially the way it impacts my relationship with food and how I overeat. I'm quite shocked by just how much power my Gremlin has. I need to come up with a powerful mantra to keep it in check.

Mantra shortlist:

This isn't helpful

Enough

You're not welcome

It's the only way I'm going to make changes and stop overeating. This is actually quite exciting. For the first time, I can see the way out. I feel lighter already.

Actions for this week:

Practise with different mantras.

Choose one.

Pam (handwritten letter, which she decides to post)

Dear Helen,

I hope you won't mind me writing to you like this out of the blue, but there's something I need to tell you and I don't know if we'll get the chance to talk in private before the holiday next week.

Before I go into it, I want to tell you what a fantastic person you are and how much I have enjoyed being your daughter-in-law for all these years. I do so hope that what I'm going to say doesn't cause any tension between us and we can carry on being good friends. Anyway, here goes.

As you know I've been struggling with my weight for a while now, ever since Charlie was born, and I'm not getting anywhere with Weight Watchers. So I decided to try something else. I'm reading a book which suggests a completely different way of dealing with it and it's made a big difference to how I think about food.

I've realised that when we go away on holiday with you I eat a lot more than usual. Much more than I need really. You are such a great cook and I know all the trouble you go to making all those lovely meals and how everyone else tucks in. But, if I'm honest, we have such big breakfasts and your teas are such feasts that I'm not very hungry at lunch and probably only need half of what I eat at dinner.

So I suppose what I am saying is that I hope you won't be offended if I don't eat everything at every meal, and if I say no to your delicious food. I do hope you understand. I know how important it is to you that we all eat together. I'd love to sit and keep you all company without eating, if I'm not hungry. Would that be ok?

Do give me a ring if you want to chat about this.

With all my love

Pammy xxxx

TAKE ACTION

Keep experimenting with your superpowers and find a way to record your progress: write, draw, publish … whatever works for you. Taking time to reflect, keeping track of how you're doing can be helpful. It's great to be able to look back and take stock of how far you've come and what's still to work on.

YOUR **ACTION** CHECKLIST

☐ **Make it official:** call it overeating

☐ **Observe yourself with curiosity:** overeat with awareness

☐ **Identify your triggers:** find out why you overeat

☐ **Lighten the load:** talk about what it's really like

☐ **Find out about your forbidden foods:** make a list

☐ **Tune in to your Gremlin:** get to know it

☐ **Tune in to your feelings:** name and acknowledge them

☐ **Tune in to your overeating body:** listen to your body talk

☐ **Pause:** for just one minute

→

☐ **Stock up:** legalise your forbidden foods

☐ **Experiment with your superpowers:** 1-minute mantra, feelings tool-kit, body talk

☐ **Record your progress:** keep experimenting and record your progress

•

CHAPTER THIRTEEN

Making it Happen

THIS IS IT. The moment you've been waiting for. The time has come to make it happen and to stop overeating. Not for ever, not from now on, just once. And then again and then again and then again. Because that's how we stop for good. One step at a time.

SO MANY WOMEN ... STOPPING ...

All these women are making it happen. They have all decided not to overeat, just once.

Alice is having a tea break with a cuppa and her favourite chocolate chip cookies. There's a big glass jar full of them on the table in front of her. She's eaten two and has enjoyed every bite. As she gets up to put her mug in the sink and the cookie jar back in the cupboard, she thinks to herself:

I could have another one. She recognises the trigger, STOPS and tunes in.

Gremlin: You could. It's fine. It's just one.

Alice: Be quiet (firm and decisive).

Gremlin: It won't spoil anything. They say you should eat your forbidden foods when you want them, so technically it's allowed.

Alice: Be quiet.

Gremlin: Just this once. You can start properly again at dinner.

Alice: BE QUIET.

Outcome

Alice puts the lid back on the biscuit jar. She's feeling triumphant.

✦

Becky is at a restaurant, towards the end of a big meal, feeling pleasantly full, dessert menu in hand. She STOPS and tunes in.

Gremlin: I want the mousse, I really want it.

Becky: I know (calm, adult, kind).

Gremlin: No, but I really want it. I really, *really* want it . . . whimper . . .

Becky: I know.

Gremlin: Pleeease, I love chocolate mousse, I never get to eat it.

Becky: I know.

Gremlin: Stop saying that, I want it. What's wrong with having pudding? Everyone else will . . . I really want it.

Becky: I know.

Gremlin: Oh, it's not fair. I want it, I really want, I can't do this. It's not working, I want it . . .

Becky: I know.

Gremlin: No, you don't know. Just this time. I'll stop tomorrow. Please . . .

Becky: I know.

The Gremlin gives up. Becky feels shaky and tearful, overwhelmed with sadness and longing. She can't cry now, not in a restaurant in front of all these people. She decides to put the feelings in her safe box and promises herself she'll open it up when she gets home. She takes a deep breath and decides to focus on her body talk. She sits up straighter in her chair, pulls back her shoulders, blinks her eyes and shakes her head softly. She takes another deep, steadying breath and lets the air out slowly through her mouth.

Outcome

Becky closes the menu and hands it back to the waiter with a smile saying: 'I'm fine, thanks. I'll just have a coffee.'

◆

Christine is walking through reception to collect her next patient. She's rummaging absentmindedly in her pocket for another jelly bean. She STOPS, takes her hand out of her pocket, turns around and walks back to her room, shuts the door and tunes in.

She recognises an overwhelming feeling of anxiety. She walks over to her dentist's chair, climbs on to it, leans back and closes her eyes. The anxiety feels like a burning ball of tension gnawing in the pit of her stomach. She decides to give herself a few minutes to acknowledge the anxiety and feel it. She tracks it as it washes through her. She feels tense and tight all over. Even her ponytail feels tight, pulling at her head. She takes out the elastic and shakes her hair loose. She takes a few slow, deep breaths, imagines the ball melting away and feels her belly softening.

Outcome

After a few more minutes, she gets up, empties the jelly beans out of her pocket and into the top drawer of her desk. She puts her hair back in a ponytail, a bit looser this time and walks back out to reception to meet her patient.

Debbie is at the petrol station again, in the queue holding two Picnic bars. There are just a couple of people in front of her waiting to pay. She looks at the bars of chocolate in her hand. She STOPS and tunes in.

Gremlin: You've picked them up now.

Debbie: Mmmh . . . (Disinterested, with a shrug. She puts the chocolate back.)

Gremlin: No, no, no. Don't put them back. You'll regret it later.

Debbie: Mmmh . . . (Shrugs.)

Gremlin: Hurry up, you're next.

Debbie: Mmmh . . . (Shrugs, still looking at the chocolate.)

Gremlin: Get them, just get them, just in case. You don't have to eat them.

Debbie: Mmmh . . . (Shrugs.)

Gremlin: There's nothing else at home. You're going to regret it. You can't, what are you going to do tonight?

Debbie: Mmmh . . . (Shrugs.)

Outcome

She turns away from the chocolate and pays for her petrol. She walks back to the car, sits in her seat and does a little jig of happiness. She's amazed. It's the first time she's ever said no to herself without feeling deprived.

◆

Emily is sitting in the car with a pack of cocktail sausages in her hands. She rips it open and stuffs one in her mouth. As she's chewing, she remembers that she promised she would interrupt herself the next time she did this. She STOPS and tunes in.

The only thing she she's aware of is a rush of anger. No, make that fury. She tunes in to her body. She's clenching her teeth and pulling back her lips. She catches herself in the rear-view mirror: there are two bright red patches on her cheeks and the tendons in her neck are sticking out. Her whole upper body is tense. She knows what she needs to do. She puts the car in gear and drives to the quiet end of the car park. And then she lets rip. She roars like a lion. She does it again, with her whole body this time. And then takes a few deep breaths and sits back in the seat. Exhausted. That felt good. That felt *really* good.

Outcome

Emily gets out of the car and throws the sausages in a bin.

✦

Fatima is standing at the fridge eating. She's about to reach for another piece of quiche. She takes a deep breath, STOPS, her hand in mid-air, and tunes in. She feels panicky.

Gremlin: Oh my God oh my God oh my God

Fatima: Shhhhhh . . . (Gentle and reassuring. She takes another deep breath and notices her panic subside just a little.)

Gremlin: I feel terrible, I can't cope. I have to eat.

Fatima: Shhhhhh . . . (She takes a deep breath, drops her shoulders, stretches her fingers, takes another deep breath and plants both feet firmly on the floor)

Gremlin: Oh God . . . Oh God . . .

Fatima: Shhhhhh . . . (Takes another deep breath)

She tunes in. She knows she's not hungry, she's eaten enough. She starts to shut the fridge door and her Gremlin starts up again.

Gremlin: No, it's not enough, it's not enough.

Fatima: Shhhhhh . . . (Takes another deep breath)

Outcome

Fatima walks back to bed, taking deep, steady breaths all the way.

✦

Grace is sitting on the sofa at home watching telly when she gets the urge to go to the kitchen for something to eat. She gets up and is making her way down the stairs to the basement when she suddenly STOPS dead in her tracks.

Grace: Oi! Fuck off! (Loud. Definitive.)

Gremlin: No. Eat!

Grace: Oi! Fuck OFF!

Gremlin: Eat for fuck's sake. I need food!

Grace: OI! FUCK. OFF!

Grace turns around and heads back up the stairs to the living room. She sits down on the sofa, takes a deep breath and tunes in. She scans her body, but comes up blank. All she is aware of is a loud buzzing in her head. All she can think of is how angry she is. Angry. Angry. Angry.

Outcome

Grace goes over to the computer and opens a new document. She starts writing. She writes about how angry she is, her fingers flying over the keyboard. She writes and writes without stopping, until she has nothing more to write. She reads over what she has written, tears welling up in her eyes as she reads certain bits, nodding at others. She saves the document in a folder called 'Rants' and then flops down on to the sofa, exhausted. Exhausted and relieved. The buzzing in her head has gone.

✦

Heather is driving home after a stressful work meeting. Somewhere at the back of her mind she knows that she's heading towards the Drive-Thru, although she hasn't acknowledged this to herself yet. As she approaches a red light, she slows the car down and slows her thoughts down too. She STOPS and tunes in.

Gremlin: Oh, stop it. This is ridiculous. You are ridiculous. I can't believe you're still at it! It's just pathetic. You tune in and then what? Realise what a hopeless, pathetic human being you are. What are you going to do with that?

Heather: STOP! (Very loud, nearly shouting.)

Gremlin: Stop what? You make me sick. You sound like some kind of schizo'. Maybe you are. You're a fat, greedy schizo'. That's what you are. Pretending to yourself that you're normal. Posting on that stupid little forum like you're normal. Don't you see? Don't you see that you're . . .

Heather: STOP! JUST STOP!

Gremlin: Stop . . . just stop (*mimicking her*). Whine, whine . . . all you can do is whi—

Heather: STOOOOOOOOOP!

Heather is aware of shaking all over. She pulls over to the kerb and puts her head in her hands, willing herself to breathe, taking in huge, ragged gulps of air.

Outcome

When she has stopped shaking and is breathing normally again she does a U-turn and drives home. When she gets home, she goes straight to her computer to post on the forum and share her success with the others.

✦

Isabelle is sitting in her room, bored again, really bored. She's staring at her computer. The screensaver appears: the words TUNE IN slide back and forth across the screen in big green letters. She watches them, debating whether to just go down to the kitchen or to have a go at tuning in. She STOPS and tunes in.

Gremlin: Go on, go down and get something. Why are you even pretending that you're not going to?

Isabelle: Piss off. (*Firm and threatening.*)

Gremlin: You can tell me to piss off all you like, you know you can't resist. Just do it and get it over with.

Isabelle: Piss off.

Gremlin: Go on. Go.

Isabelle: Piss off.

Gremlin: This isn't going to work. You can't do it. Just eat.

Isabelle feels trapped. Her Gremlin is right. It's not going to work. She decides to try another tack. What feeling is she aware of? She clicks the screen to life and goes to the document with the worksheet on it. She scans the feelings column. Nothing. She doesn't feel any of them. This is hopeless. Is that her Gremlin again? PISS OFF. Ok, Body talk, then. She tunes in. She's very still. Very still. Not moving, breathing very shallowly. Her mouth is shut tight.

She's squeezing the mouse very tightly with her hand. She's pulling her belly in. It feels like she's stopping herself from doing something. She scans the feelings list again. Angry. It suddenly jumps off the page at her. She's angry. Really? Why? Why doesn't matter, remember. What now? Use one of the tools. She grabs her Biro and starts scrawling on a piece of paper. She just keeps dragging the pen across the page furiously, digging into the paper, over and over, until it's almost completely covered with angry black lines. She stares at it and takes a deep breath.

Outcome

She feels calmer. The urge to eat has passed.

◆

Jane is at the supermarket, standing in the crisps aisle. She picks up a multipack of Walkers cheese and onion and, as she puts it in her basket, she jumps as if she's received an electric shock. Seeing the bag in her basket has reminded her of tuning in. She STOPS and cocks her head, listening out for her Gremlin and sure enough:

Gremlin: I'm soooo tired. Just a little treat. I won't eat them all.

Jane: Yeah, yeah, yeah. Yadda, yadda, yadda.

Gremlin: But I am. I'm exhausted.

Jane: Yeah, yeah, yeah. Yadda, yadda, yadda.
Jane decides she's bored of her Gremlin and tunes in to her body. What's it *like* when she's tired? Head pounding, eyes burning, everything heavy: eyelids, shoulders, belly, buttocks all feel like they are dragging downward. Jane thinks that if

she could, she'd sit down right here, right now, in the middle of the supermarket and have a good cry. She remembers her lovely, gem-studded safe box and decides to contain the sadness until she gets home. Then she remembers that Pete will be back from the park with the children and decides to hold on to the tears until she gets to the car.

Outcome

Jane puts the crisps back on the shelf, pays for her shopping and goes to sit in her car where she sobs her heart out and feels really sorry for herself for five minutes. She drives home feeling refreshed and curiously rested.

✦

Kate is on a business trip. She's sitting in a restaurant on her own, eating roast sea bass and spinach. She's been eyeing the bread basket longingly since she sat down, debating whether to have a piece.

Gremlin: Oh, you are such a fraud. Can't you just make up your mind and stick to your decision. What's the point of making all these promises, if you're just going to break them the minute temptation comes your way. Get a grip, for goodness sake.

Kate: That's not helpful. (*Matter of fact.*)

Gremlin: If you're going to have it, just have it. You always do.

Kate: That's not helpful.

Gremlin: So what? It's true.

Kate: That's not helpful.

Gremlin: You might as well – you'll only end up eating the biscuits back in the room like last time.

Kate: That's. Not. Helpful.

Gremlin: Maybe not, but you can't deny that's what you did.

Kate: That's. Not. Helpful.

The Gremlin goes quiet. Kate waits for a moment, listening out for more. She breathes. Nothing comes. She looks at the bread and asks herself why she wants it *so* much. The answer comes back like a flash. 'Because I *can't* have it.' If she has it, she won't feel good. It just doesn't agree with her. But hold on a minute, actually she *can* – she *can* put it in her mouth. Nothing is stopping her. But she doesn't *want* to. She wants to feel good more than she wants to eat the bread. She's making a choice. 'I'm choosing not to have it,' she says, under her breath. 'I am making a choice; this is *my* choice.'

Outcome

Kate leaves the table, the bread basket untouched. She feels calm and very proud of herself. It feels good to know that she always has a choice.

✦

Leila is in the kitchen, making a cup of tea, waiting for the kettle to boil. She's got loads to do and she wishes she could add an extra few hours to the day so she could get through it all. Her eyes hover over the biscuit tin and the usual debate starts up. She hears herself think and decides to STOP and tune in. Her Gremlin is at it again. Will it ever let up?

Gremlin: Just put a few on a plate, there's nothing wrong with that.

Leila: Yeah, except I'm not hungry and I know what will happen – a few will lead to the whole pack.

Gremlin: No, it'll be fine. Things are much better now.

Leila is about to argue back when she remembers her mantra.

Leila: I don't have time for this. Quiet. (Authoritative and dismissive.)

Gremlin: Ok, so just take the biscuits and go back to your desk.

Leila: I don't have time for this. Quiet.

Gremlin: Just a few maybe?

Leila: I don't have time for this. Quiet.

Outcome

The kettle boils, she makes herself a cup of tea and goes back to her desk – biscuitless and feeling smug.

✦

Natasha is at her nephew's birthday party. Her sister has put on the most amazing spread. All their childhood favourites. She wants one of EVERYTHING.

Gremlin: Oh wow, look at all this stuff. Have one of each.

Natasha: Whatever. (Sounding like a teenager.)

Gremlin: Oh boring! Go on. Who cares? You only live once.

Natasha: Whatever.

Gremlin: Fuck it, go on. Come on. It's ok. I really don't care. I don't give a shit.

Natasha: Whatever.

Gremlin: Am I serious? Am I really going to do this? I don't think so. It's a party, for God's sake. I'm supposed to, it's a party. Everyone else is going to.

Natasha: Whatever.

Gremlin: Oh my God. I'm serious. I think I really mean it.

Natasha: Whatever, whatever, whatever.

Outcome

Natasha looks at the table, laden with goodies and takes her time. She settles on a few delicate-looking little sandwiches (no crusts), a fabulous piece of fudge cake and a couple of her sister's homemade jammy dodgers, her absolute favourites. She's about to add a little pot of lime jelly and she stops; she puts it back on the table and walks away muttering, 'Whatever' under her breath. She knows there will be many more birthdays – her nephew is only four!

✦

Olivia is at her company's Christmas dinner. She is sitting at a table where everyone is chatting away, with a plateful of food in front of her. As she picks up her fork again, she looks down at her hands and sees that her watch is on the wrong wrist. And then she remembers. She remembers that she has come prepared. She STOPS, opens her bag and pretends to be looking for something as she reads the instructions on the little card she put in there earlier. She tunes in.

Thoughts: You don't belong here. You have nothing to say. Eat this; it will help, give you something to do with yourself.

Feeling: Dread

Body talk: Slumped in the chair, shoulders hunched forward, face flushed, mouth turned downward, hot and sweaty, clothes too tight, breathing shallow.

Olivia scans the card and considers her options. She knows her Gremlin won't let up if she listens, and she can't think of anything she can do here with the dread. She decides to reorganise her body talk.

She sits up straighter in her chair, plants both feet firmly on the floor and moves her shoulders around, trying to find a position where they feel comfortable: neither hunched forward nor pulled back. She wills her lips into a slight smile, unbuttons her cardigan a little and focuses on sending her breath all the way down into her belly. She shifts a little in her seat, to get comfortable in this unfamiliar position, breathing slowly and steadily all the time.

She tunes in again. She realises that her Gremlin has gone silent. She shivers slightly, as she imagines the black goo retreating, slithering away somewhere dark and cold, waiting, watching. The dread has subsided and now she's just feeling a little anxious. It's ok, she thinks, I can do anxious.

Outcome

Olivia pushes her plate away and turns round to her neighbour. She takes a deep breath and says: 'How long have you worked here?'

✦

Pam is at the office, sitting at her desk. She gets up and makes her way slowly to the vending machine, caught up in her thoughts. As she drops the coins distractedly into the slot, she comes out of her reverie and shakes her head. No, she reminds herself. I don't want to overeat. She STOPS and tunes in.

Nothing. Blank. She can't focus. She has no idea what she's thinking, apart from not knowing what she's thinking. She doesn't feel anything in particular, however hard she tries, and she couldn't say anything about her body except that she's standing up and her heart is beating quite fast. She's not sure what this last piece of information means.

Outcome

After a moment like this, she decides to go back to her desk. She logs on to the forum and starts to write a post about what's just happened. As she writes, she realises that she has been worrying all day about going to dinner at a friend's. She writes about being unable to say 'No' to her friend's lovely food. About not wanting to offend her, about how she overeats every time she goes out to dinner. She writes about her reproachful granny, how she shames her into eating with a million trite sayings. When she's done, she feels relieved and notices her heart is beating normally again. She stays away from the vending machine for the rest of the afternoon.

HOW TO MAKE IT HAPPEN

Reading this book alone is unlikely to change your relationship with food and stop you overeating. Very, very unlikely. In fact, we may as well be bold and just say it won't.

All change requires action

If you want a different experience, it's up to you to *do* something different, to take action. You don't have to *try hard*, you don't have to push yourself or force yourself. What you do have to do is take ACTION. One step, and then another and then another. What you have to do is to have a go – do something different *once*, experiment and then experiment again. Taking action leads to changing behaviours. Taking action and doing something different will open you up to a different experience. So as well as reading this book, use the information in it to experiment. Do something – pick any part of it that appeals to you and take action.

Where to start

Whatever you start with, the way in is through tuning in and then choosing to do something different. So you don't necessarily have to go through your Gremlin, feelings and body talk – use whatever you think will work best, whatever you need in the moment. It may change from one time to the next.

And it doesn't matter which tool you use either – whether it's your mantra or one from the feelings tool-kit or reorganising your body talk. Keep tuning in and keep experimenting.

Here's a quick reminder of the tools:

1-minute mantra

Remember to stay with it, to keep repeating it until your Gremlin retreats, gives up and goes quiet.

Don't deviate from your mantra, remember, no discussions or arguments with your Gremlin. Repetition and perseverance are key. Give yourself at least one minute. Your Gremlin is unlikely to roll over and give up without a fight.

The feelings tool-kit

FEEL IT

In a safe place

Set a time

Feel the feeling

EXPLORE IT

Draw

Journal

Write a letter
(for your eyes only)

SHARE IT

Post on the Forum

Speak to someone
who understands
and knows how to
listen

CONTAIN IT

Put it in your
safe box

Commit to
opening it up again

Reorganising your body talk

Remember to start with your breath and your posture and then scan the rest of your body. Include your face, internal sensations and how you feel in your clothes. Then make a conscious decision to change something about the way you are holding yourself.

Keep practising

The more you practise stopping, and the more you use any one (or several) of these tools when you stop – however gradually – the better you will get at doing it. Eventually, you won't always have to consciously think about it. By doing it over and over again, overeating stops being the best option.

IF YOU'RE STUCK

You may come up with 100 reasons why you can't stop: why it's too difficult, too risky, too crazy. You may find you forget, avoid or make excuses not to use any of these tools. This is your Gremlin talking. Gremlins don't like change. They want everything to stay just as it is. They like the status quo. So, if you notice yourself thinking:

✦ I can't do this

✦ it's too hard

✦ it will never work

✦ this will work for other people, but not for me

✦ I shouldn't do this

✦ I don't want to

✦ I'm scared

✦ this is terrifying

✦ this is a load of rubbish

+ I don't know how to do it

+ why can't I do it now, I was doing fine last week . . .

. . . it's either your Gremlin talking or you need more time in the **GET READY** section. As a rule of thumb, if it's keeping you from doing something you really want to do (and we are assuming here that you *really* want to stop overeating), and you know you've been practising and pausing, then it's probably your Gremlin at work – and now you know exactly how to deal with it. You are in charge. You decide. Until you have a go, you won't know.

SUPPORT YOURSELF

We've seen over and over again that support can make the difference between failure and success. It doesn't matter how you support yourself, the important thing is to find a way of doing something that works for you.

APPRECIATE YOURSELF

It's so easy to focus on the overeating we are *still* doing, the actions we *haven't* done, the things we are struggling with. We beat ourselves up for not doing enough and generally give ourselves a hard time. Shift the focus. Every time you take even a tiny little step, every time you experiment with one of the actions, even if it doesn't go perfectly to plan, appreciate yourself. Appreciate yourself for taking action and plan to do it again.

DON'T TRY

If you only *think* about using the tools in this book or just *try* to use them, nothing will change.

Trying means *thinking* about doing something, without actually doing it. *Trying* means promising to ourselves that we will do something without actually doing it. *Trying* means thinking that we *should* do something, when our heart is not really in it or we are not quite ready and then forgetting or finding reasons why we *can't do it.*

Trying means doing something without engaging with it; following rules, going through the motions without questioning, without challenging, without examining, without taking responsibility for or ownership of our actions.

You don't have to succeed in order for it to count as taking action. You may think that you are only trying when you experiment with one of the actions and don't quite manage it or it doesn't have the outcome you were hoping for first time. Let's imagine you are learning to ride a bike. You start by getting on, putting your feet on the pedals and moving your legs round, etc., you may not manage to ride the bike very far, but you've done more than just think about doing it. If you get on the bike, if you're sitting on the saddle and you are moving your legs around, you *are* riding it, not just trying. You may not be riding it successfully, you may not have mastered the art of peddling and staying balanced quite yet, you may not even get very far, but you are not trying – you are doing it, you are learning how to ride it. You *are* riding the bike.

Don't *try*.

Take action. **Just Do It**.

TAKE ACTION

- **Make it happen.** Plan to STOP, just once.

- **Plan it in advance.** It could be the next time you overeat or on a specific day or in a specific situation when you know you are likely to overeat.

- **Remember you can STOP at any point.** Before you overeat or while you're doing it.

EPILOGUE

·

Some Time in the Future

IT'S A SUNNY AND CRISP Saturday morning in central London. The hotel is one of those grand old dames which was once chic and is now fraying a little at the edges. The room is huge and yet quite intimate. At the far end, fifteen women are sitting in a circle. The circle is interrupted by two empty chairs separated by a flipchart and a little table sporting a tiny vase with a slender pink tulip. Some of the women are chatting, some are staring out of the window or at their hands. A few are writing in journals or tapping on their phones.

The door at the far end opens and Sophie walks in, followed by Audrey. They cross the room and sit down on the empty chairs. As they settle, they take a moment to look around the group, smiling and looking into the eyes of each woman in turn, acknowledging them for being here.

Sophie breaks the silence: 'Thank you all for coming today. It's great to have you all here.'

'Yes, welcome. Thank you all for making it here. Some of you have come a really long way. It's lovely to meet you all,' says Audrey.

Sophie continues: 'Before we get into the nitty gritty of the workshop, we'd love to hear from you. We'd like you to introduce yourselves. You've all read the book and we know you've been putting it all into practice. We'd like you to take a moment now, to think about what's changed since you started. What have you been doing differently? What have you noticed? And what's your work in progress? What needs more time and attention? Take a few minutes now to think about it. You can make some notes in your journals, if you like, and when you're ready, we'll hear from whoever would like to go first.

In the meantime, Audrey gets up and writes the following on the flipchart in large purple marker pen:

Introductions

What's changed?

What's work in progress?

Anything else?

'So,' Sophie says after a few minutes, 'who would like to go first?'

There's a moment of silence as the women look at each other nervously. Everyone is holding back. Those who want to dive in and can't wait to get started, don't want to look pushy. And those who want a hole to open up under their chairs and swallow them up, wish someone else would go first, because they certainly won't.

Pam straightens slightly in her chair and gives a nervous cough:

'I'll go first. I don't mind. Someone's got to! So, um, yes.
Well, I'm **Pam**, and I have to say that quite a lot has
changed. I suppose the biggest thing is how aware I am of
everything now. And it's true that sometimes just knowing
what I'm doing means I don't do it the same way. I've been
overeating less and less. It's astonishing really. I mean
specifically what I've understood is just how much my
mother and my grandmother influenced the way I think
about food. They lived through the war and rationing and
we never had much money, so they were always going on
about waste and finishing what's on your plate, and eating
what you're given and all that sort of thing. I don't think I
was ever once asked what I *wanted* to eat. And it's another
generation isn't it? All those rules about being polite and
never refusing food and not making a fuss and eating what
everyone else is eating.

'Well, anyway . . . when I started to tune in and
discovered my Gremlin – I've called her the reproachful
granny – I realised just how much of the eating I did was
triggered by those thoughts. It also means I overeat less in
other moments too. Somehow, it's like I've been living in a
fog and now I can see.'

Pam pauses and takes a deep breath.

'Anyway, as for the work in progress, it's the same really. I
know that eating something so as not to offend someone
isn't what I want to be doing, but on some level, I sort of
agree that it's nicer not to offend people, so I'm grappling
with that one sometimes. I've also realised that I am

anxious a lot of the time and haven't found the best way of managing it yet. I keep on looking at the feelings tool-kit and telling myself I'll have a go tomorrow and then I don't. So, that's work in progress.'

She sighs and glances at the flipchart.

'So, ummm, anything else? Well, nothing except that I wanted to say how lovely it is to be here with all of you!'

She turns to look at Sophie:

'Was that ok?'

'Thank you, Pam. That was fine. Who would like to go next?'

Jane takes a deep breath and pushes herself forward on her seat. Her face is flushed. 'I'll go next,' she says.

'Uh, yes, hello, my name's **Jane**. Uh, where do I start? Oh yes, so what's changed? Well . . . I don't know where to start, really. I was thinking about it in the car on the way here. Sometimes, it feels like nothing has changed really. I'm still exhausted most of the time, I still eat when the kids are napping and I still sometimes have two dinners. But if I think about it, actually lots has changed. It's just that it's little things, so I forget that the bigger picture is actually very different. Sometimes I actually nap with the children now. I can't believe I was so tired and never did anything about it. I just sat there and ate.'

She laughs.

'And now I lie down for an hour while they sleep and I feel so much better. And I hardly ever eat at nap times any more. I mean I know I said I do, but actually, when I think about it, it's so much less than it used to be. Oh, and I catch myself eating mindlessly all the time now. I've gotten really good at it. Seriously, I can't believe how much I used to eat without really admitting it to myself. So that's good. And then last week, I did something I've never done before: I had tea with the children. I actually sat down with them and ate shepherd's pie and peas and jelly. And when Pete came home I sat with him while he ate and just chatted. I don't think he even noticed. So that's really good. Anyway, as I said: the little things all add up. I feel better. I've even had my hair cut. I just don't feel so awful all the time any more. I don't know if it's because I'm eating less or if I'm eating less because I don't feel awful, but whatever it is, it works.'

She beams around the group of women and then frowns.

'I don't want to sound boastful and like it's all fixed, though. I mean, I do still overeat sometimes. And also, I'm finding the whole forbidden-foods thing with kids impossible, so I'm not really doing that – and I know I should because that's the stuff I overeat on a lot. Oh, and another thing, which is sort of "work in progress", but also "anything else". I've decided to train as a baby-massage therapist. It means I've got to get childcare for a few hours a week, so I don't know, but next year, if my mum can help. I know that's not about overeating, but actually I never would have had the courage to go for it before, so it is really.'

'Thanks Jane.' There's a moment of silence. Sophie and Audrey look around the circle of women and smile encouragingly.

'Ok, I'll go next. Erm, what's changed? Oh, sorry, I'm **Natasha**.'

She takes a deep breath and carries on talking excitedly.

'I know this sounds a bit cheesy, but everything has; this has literally changed my life. I used to think about food all the time. Honestly, if I wasn't actually eating, I was thinking about what I could eat and when I'd have it. I think the thing that's been the most amazing is allowing myself to eat whatever I want. Oh and realising that I'm ok with my body – that I quite like the way I look. I always thought that I needed to lose weight, mainly because you're not supposed to feel ok if you're not slim, at least that's what I used to think. If I'm honest, that's why I picked up the book in the first place. I thought if I could stop overeating, then I'd lose weight. But the thing is, now that I'm more relaxed about what I eat, because I let myself have the things I want, you know, all those things we cut out when we're on diets.'

She pauses for a just a moment and looks around the room.

'Well, at least, *I* do. Well, now that I just go ahead and have them, they've become less special, or something like that. So I end up eating them less. And, I never thought I would *ever* say anything like this, but sometimes I don't even want them, and I don't have them at all. Er, I've lost my thread a bit . . . oh yes, since I've stopped feeling guilty and telling myself I can't have this and I shouldn't have that, I've actually lost a bit of weight. And it's really odd, but I'm not that fussed. I just feel so different. It's as if someone has lifted this huge, big boulder off my shoulders. I don't feel guilty any more, I don't stress about food any more.

'What else? Oh yes, work in progress? Well, I think sometimes I just don't bother to use the mantra and I still let my Gremlin take charge. It takes quite an effort to stay with it and I think sometimes, especially when I'm at a party or out to dinner or something like that, I can get distracted or I just forget. But that's not all the time. I do use the mantra quite a lot and it really works – mine's "Whatever" and it really does the trick. I think it's coz it's not too serious or anything. I'd love to know what everyone else's is. Anyway, that's me. Is that it?'

She glances at the flipchart.

'Anything else? Erm, no, not for now. I think that's it, really.'

'Shall I go next? Hi, I'm **Debbie**. I can really relate to what you were saying, Natasha. I can't believe what a difference it's made to legalise my forbidden foods. I've been cooking more and just *enjoying* food so much more. I feel a bit nervous admitting this, but I used to . . . '

She hesitates and when she speaks again her voice is quieter, more tentative:

'I used to buy a bar of chocolate, even two or three or even more, every time I stopped at the petrol station. And I used to eat it in the car. I don't think I even enjoyed it much, which sounds crazy. Sometimes, I used to stop at the petrol station just *so* I could buy the chocolate.'

She looks down at the floor and then around the room at the other women.

'I even went down there really late at night to get chocolate, sometimes. But yesterday, when I stopped to fill up, I just looked at the chocolate and I found myself thinking: I *could* buy one, but I don't really want one. So I didn't. That may not sound like a big deal, but it's just amazing, really amazing. It's not that I don't ever eat chocolate. I do. And I've got lots of it at home now, so if I want some, I just sit down and have it. I just feel so much less worried about it all now.

'What's my work in progress? Well, there's something about meals out, I think. Last weekend, I went out to dinner and I just couldn't stop myself having pudding. I wasn't hungry for it, really, but it just looked so lovely. I don't know why I didn't tune in. I think in a way, I knew that if I tuned in, I probably wouldn't eat it and I wanted to. So I suppose that's something I need to work on a bit more. I'm still not very good at the body-talk thing. I just can't quite work out what I'm doing, even when I really tune in and concentrate. It's a bit tricky, really. But I'd like to get the hang of it, so I'll keep trying.'

She smiles at Sophie and Audrey.

'I mean, not *trying* – having a go, practising!'

She laughs.

Sophie smiles back at her. 'Thanks, Debbie.'

'Hiya. My name's **Fatima**. It's so inspiring listening to you all, but I feel like I haven't really changed much. I mean, I have done *one* thing that's brilliant, I suppose. I've stopped dieting. I mean completely. My dad doesn't know, though.'

She pauses.

'It's really funny, isn't it? Because I know some of you'

She looks around the room and smiles at Debbie

– 'from the forum. And I might even have spoken to some of you without knowing, if you haven't got your photo on there. It's so amazing to be here, all together. So, anyway, some of you know about my dad. He's a doctor and he's *so* controlling. He thinks I should be on a diet and he goes on and on about my weight. After I read the book, I decided that was it. It wasn't working anyway, so I've stopped starving myself during the day. I'm not following his plans any more. But, I don't, like, quite have the courage to tell him. To confront him. He'd go ballistic, if he found out. I just don't say anything, but I'm eating normally in the day.'

She frowns, thoughtfully.

'D'you know, I didn't realise until I said it that I really *am* eating more normally in the daytime. Like, I'm not trying to survive on less than 900 calories a day any more. I don't raid the fridge when they've all gone to bed either, but I still end up pigging out on chocolate in my bedroom sometimes. I just wish I could eat what I want. If he'd just leave me to do my own thing. Yeah, I wish. I think the legalising food thing is what I want to do, so that's my work in progress, I guess. I just think that would make such a difference, but I can't have all the stuff I want at home, I just can't. I'm not sure how to work it out at the moment. The thing is, even though I'm not dieting, I haven't put on any weight, which is funny really. Well, maybe not. I suppose I wasn't really sticking to the diet, anyway. Well, that's me.'

'Thank you, Fatima. So, who'd like to go next?'

'Yeah, I'll go next. Hi, I'm **Isabelle – Izzy**. Yeah, I'm doing pretty well, actually. I know some of you from the forum will know about the bulimia; I've never talked about it before like that. The college have organised for me to see a counsellor and it's quite cool. I like that she is telling me not to stop purging until I'm ready. It fits in with Beyond Temptation and the not stopping overeating. But to be honest, I'm throwing up less anyway. I mean, I know I can always do it, and I always think about doing it, but I have had a few times when I didn't. I don't know if I'll ever be able to stop; sometimes it doesn't feel like I can, but I really want to and the counsellor says that that's the most important bit. I chucked my noxious boyfriend. I've gone on and on about this on the forum. So now he's gone I feel so much better. That and the counselling for working on my bingeing . . . it's been a really cool year, actually. I just feel better about myself, I'm having more fun and I think I've lost some weight. These jeans used to be quite tight and I need a belt now.

'Ummm what else? I don't sneak food any more. If I fancy a biscuit after dinner, I go down and sit there and eat it in front of my mum, and I have lunch at the cafeteria at college when I'm hungry, even if Peggy and the others don't. I don't care. Anyway, work in progress is the bulimia, of course, and that kind of goes with the overeating because it's the same thing, you know, like yin and yang. It's really cool because now I know what to do to stop overeating, I feel there is some hope that I'll be able to stop throwing up too. Yeah, that's me, really. Great to put faces to names, by the way.'

'I'm ok to go next. I'm **Becky**.'

She glances at the flipchart.

'What's changed?' She looks nervously around the room and fiddles with her pen. 'It's been a bit of a rollercoaster for me. I've had some good days and then some days where it just feels as though nothing is ever going to change. Well, maybe that's just me being negative. I have been using the mantra and I've been tuning in and reorganising my body, and when I do it, it does make a difference. I have actually been able to stop eating, even when I really like the taste and I'm enjoying it. So I *can* do it, which I didn't believe I could at the beginning. It takes a lot of effort, though. Not just plain sailing. It feels like I take two steps forward and then one step back. Is that normal?'

She glances at Sophie and then Audrey, looking for reassurance. She sees some of the other women nodding and starts speaking again.

'I think I was hoping for a magic wand. I've spent so long trying to sort this out that sometimes, I don't want to work at it, I don't want to make the effort – I just want it to happen. Reading the book is ok, but when it comes to taking action, that's my work in progress I think. When I do interrupt myself, I can actually stop. So I need to do it more. I need to stop resisting doing it and just do it. That's it, isn't it? That's what it boils down to for me.'

'Right. I'm **Kate**. Hello.'

Her voice is tight, she sits upright in her chair.

'It's a bit different for me. It's all been rather complicated.
It's because I'm intolerant to dairy; I have been since I was
a child. So I knew that before I started this, before I bought
the book. I wasn't really sure if it would work for someone
like me because I really *shouldn't* eat dairy – I feel very ill
when I do, which can make things very awkward, eating out
and that sort of thing. Then I was told to avoid wheat and
sugar as well. It made sense, of course, and having a healthy
diet is very important and they really aren't very good for
you, are they? Wheat and sugar, I mean. I'm so sorry, I know
there isn't time for the whole story, but it's important, just so
you understand. I hope I'm not taking up too much time.
I know I haven't talked about what's changed yet.'

She looks over at Sophie for reassurance.

'It's fine, Kate. Take your time.'

'Well, what I've realised is that the main problem was trying
to stop eating wheat and sugar *completely*. I thought doing it
properly, cutting them out, would be the easiest way. But the
more I tried to avoid them, the more I seemed to eat them.
It's not logical at all, but that's what kept happening. I kept
promising myself that I would stop, but it was impossible.
Wheat and sugar are everywhere, well certainly wheat is.
And I have to admit that I do like some things with wheat
and sugar in them. I genuinely don't like junk-type foods, but
things like good-quality puddings or a croissant from time to
time . . . I've been experimenting and keeping a log. It's been

very helpful. What I found out was that when I tried to resist eating a pudding, for example, I usually ended up giving in. But not only that – afterwards, just to make it even worse, I would have more of that kind of thing, usually biscuits or something. It was so stressful and hard, trying to hold back. I think when I felt I'd messed it up, I just made myself mess it up properly. Do you know what I mean? So that's been the main change for me: it's letting myself have some pudding or a croissant or a piece of cake when I really want it and not feeling bad about it. Not seeing it as a failure, which is what I was doing before. What I noticed was that my Gremlin kept telling me I'd messed up and that I was useless and would never manage it. Now, when I just have the cake, or you know, whatever it is, I can eat it and not feel guilty. It's been rather a turning point. I don't do it too often, but just knowing that it's all right to have some, when I go out or something, means I don't end up overeating at home in secret.

'Sometimes, I do catch my Gremlin giving me a hard time about it and that's when I remind it – myself, really – that it's not helpful for me to be extreme and to try to be perfect. And then when I have it like that, I don't mess it all up by eating biscuits or anything else. It's fine just to have the thing I want. So it really has been working very well. I think I used to tell myself that if I was sensible I wouldn't eat them at all, but I'm starting to change my mind a bit about that now. It is hard sometimes, so that's my challenge: not to feel guilty and not to try to be too perfect, with my diet, that is.'

She stops and looks a little edgy, stiffening, biting the inside of her cheek.

'That's it, I think.'

'Thanks Kate. Whoever's ready can go next.'

'I'm **Leila**. The first thing I want to say is that I'm really glad
I'm here. I wasn't going to come. When I got the email, I just
thought it wouldn't be for me really, but then I reckoned that
might be my Gremlin.'

She stops, looking around the room with a smile.

'I heard it loud and clear, prattling on about it being a waste
of time and money, insisting that I've got far too much to do
to spend a day with a bunch of women – no offence! – just
talking about all this stuff. I shut him up and booked before
I could change my mind. So here I am. I felt really bad when
you said how hard it's been for you, Becky.'

She tilts her head and gives Becky a sympathetic smile.

'It's just been so straightforward for me. I realised pretty
quickly that eating was my way of having a break, like
punctuating my day. I work from home. Anyway, it's been an
absolute revelation to tell my Gremlin to be quiet and get
on with my life. I love it because I'm telling it to be quiet all
the time. Not just for overeating. I know this might sound
obvious, but work is so much easier when I don't give myself
a hard time all day. For me, the work in progress is about
taking more breaks, proper ones. Ones which don't involve
going to the kitchen for the biscuit tin.'

She laughs and carries on:

'I'd like to have a proper lunch break every day, rather than
eating at my desk. I'm not quite there yet. Some days, I still

end up with a sandwich at the computer, but I'm getting there. It's really great.'

She looks at Sophie and Audrey.

'Thank you so much. I'm really glad I came and I'm looking forward to the rest of the day. Oh, and there is another thing. We had some friends over to dinner the other night and I'd cooked a lovely meal. When they left, I realised that I was really full, but I didn't feel guilty. It was all so delicious – even if I say so myself – and I enjoyed every bite. I know I didn't really need the pudding, but I just wanted it. That's ok, isn't it? Overeating sometimes, just because it's all so good and I want to? I really didn't feel bad about it and I didn't tell myself I'd have to be extra careful the next day or anything like that, and I know it's not something I'm going to do every day, so it felt all right. That's all.'

'I'll go next. My name's **Alice**. I think the most important thing for me – the thing that's changed the most – is how I am with feelings. It was a bit of a shock to realise just how anxious I feel a lot of the time. I don't think I realised before I started this. When I do the tuning in, I usually feel anxious. Sometimes I know why and sometimes I have no idea. I've been working on that a lot. The things that have been the most helpful are the body talk and the mantra, and it's true that when I tune in and notice I'm all tense and tight and I reorganise my body like it says in the book, I feel less anxious. I've been feeling more relaxed generally which has been really, well, *really* nice.

'I can't quite bring myself to go out and buy loads of my forbidden foods. I do know it's a good idea and it's really reassuring to hear that you've managed it.'

She looks over at Natasha and then Debbie.

'I just can't quite bring myself to do the stocking up yet. I'm letting myself have things I want more though, and that's been good.'

She is silent for a moment.

'I was just thinking back, remembering what it was like before. I worried about food and my weight all the time, literally. You know what I mean? And now I don't. Not in the same way at all. I feel so much more relaxed about it all. I think someone else said that, didn't they?'

She looks around the room, several women are nodding.

'I'm just going to keep doing more of the same. It's all work in progress, as far as I'm concerned. Thanks.'

There's a pause. Everyone looks around, expectantly.

'I'll go next if there's no one else who wants to. Hello everyone. I'm **Christine**. It's been fascinating sitting here listening to all of you. When I first got here, I felt so self-conscious. I wanted to run away. I know that people look at me and think she's thin, it's all right for her, she must be sorted. And I have to say, I work pretty hard at projecting that image. But then listening to everyone has reminded me that, actually, we are all the same. It's not about being thin or fat, it's about overeating, isn't it? And I do loads of that.

'So what has changed? Well, I think the best thing has to be the jelly-bean jar at work. I went out and bought a massive glass jar and filled it with jelly beans. It looks amazing. I ate loads for a while, I couldn't help it. And then one day, I realised I hadn't even looked at them for days. Days. Oh, and now I stop work early one day a week. Last patient at four, so I'm home by five-thirty. I cook dinner and everything. It's brilliant. I go out for lunch too. Proper lunch, with whoever is around. It really breaks up the day and I just don't eat all afternoon. I'm having so much less crap these days. It's really brilliant.

'I think what I've liked doing the best is the body talk. I've got back into skating – gave up years ago, you know, too busy – and I'm really enjoying that, it's brilliant. Uh . . . work in progress . . . well, really going back to what I said at the beginning, I don't talk about this stuff with anyone because most of them don't get it. I've looked at the forum and I read stuff on there, but I've never posted. I had to drag myself here today. You know, I'd like to spend more time with people like you guys, it's brilliant. So, yeah, thanks.'

'Hi, I'm **Emily**. This is going to sound really stupid.'

Emily is talking quickly, not really looking at anyone.

'I've stopped being veggie. I was vegetarian for, oh, ten years? No, twelve. And now I'm not. It's doing this that really helped me realise that I didn't want to be and that I was overeating loads because I wasn't eating meat. Does that make sense? My husband feels so strongly about it and I just went veggie when we got together, but my heart wasn't in it. And it wasn't just eating the meat in secret, which I did a lot. I think I was so angry about the hiding, and I felt so bad and guilty, that I ate just to block it all out, sometimes. It's a bit mad, I know. So I decided to tell him. It's incredible because

I thought he'd be really upset or angry, but he wasn't. He was really cool about it and said he understood. I could have done it years ago. Oh well. Hey ho. It's like I've never been veggie at all and I feel so much more, well, normal.

'On the things to work on, the work-in-progress bit, I've started eating crisps in the car again or other stuff, so I think I need to start looking at the other reasons why I overeat. It wasn't just the veggie thing, which is a shame.'

She smiles sheepishly.

'Listening to all of you has been really helpful because I can identify with so much of what you've said. I think I eat when I'm pissed off or when I'm bored, so I need to tune in more. And I think I need to, I don't know . . . reach out more or something like that. Hearing some of you talk about the forum, it sounds really supportive, so I'm going to have a look. I don't think I'm the forum type, but having met you all makes a difference, I think. Anyway. That's it from me.'

Olivia, Grace and Heather look at each other. Heather shifts around uncomfortably in her seat. When she starts talking, her voice is only just above a whisper.

'Sorry,'

She says, as her eyes tear up.

'I get very emotional when I am the centre of attention. It's silly, I know, but I can't help it.'

Someone passes her a box of tissues and she grabs a few, gratefully. She sits up a little straighter and looks around her.

'Sorry, my name's **Heather**. It's really lovely to be here. I'm sorry I'm such a mess. I'm not always like this. So anyway, sorry, I need to answer the question, don't I? What's changed? Ummmm, ummmm. Sorry, I can't seem to get hold of my thoughts.'

She stops, takes a deep breath and straightens up in her chair a little.

'Ok, what's changed? Well, I haven't been doing much, but I have been thinking a lot. I know that this is the best way, it makes so much sense, but . . . I don't know, I've been resisting doing the actions, you know the pause and actual stopping. I mean I did at the beginning. I paused quite a few times and even didn't overeat a few times when I decided. But . . . '

She starts to cry again.

'Sorry, sorry. It's just that I've realised that if I stop overeating, I'll probably lose weight and I don't know who I am if I'm not fat. But I want to stop so much. How can I *want* to be fat?'

She sobs and buries her face in the tissues.

'It sounds to me like you've been taking a lot of action, Heather. Pausing and stopping are just two of the steps. You've been doing a lot of Gremlin work too, thinking about what you have to lose,' says Audrey.

'Yes,' adds Sophie. 'And it can be scary to change something we've been doing for a long time.'

Heather sits up straighter again and wipes her face.

'Yes, yes, I can't believe how horrible I am to myself . . . all
the time, really horrible. I still don't really know sometimes
if it's me or my Gremlin speaking. Sometimes I think it's him
wanting me to stay fat, but I don't know . . . it's also what
I really think. I'm scared of not being fat. Is that me or my
Gremlin? Sorry, oh sorry. I'm not doing this properly, am I?
Anyway, I suppose what I've talked about is what's work in
progress. What's changed is that I'm thinking about it and
talking about it now, and I don't feel so alone with it any
more. The ladies on the forum are all so kind. I've never
been able to talk like this before – to anyone.' She starts
sniffing again.

'Sorry, for going on and blubbing like this. And thank you
for all being so lovely.'

Grace looks at Olivia.

'My turn? Hello. I'm **Grace**. I think that everything everyone
has said today is true for me in some way. I realised earlier
that I've been nodding my head the whole time. So, yes,
a bit of what everyone has said, really. Also, for me, what's
changed is that I still overeat, but in a completely different
way. I know it sounds awful, but it's like I plan to overeat.
Not in a bad way. It's just that before I was like a zombie, like
never realising that I was doing it. I mean, I knew, of course,
I knew – but I never really admitted it to myself. Now, when
I overeat, I do it deliberately. I don't try to stop. I just enjoy
it. I love eating in front of the telly, but now I'll get a proper
tray and put lots of nice things in bowls, you know like olives
and cheese and crisps and peanuts. I'm still overeating, but I

don't really care. Oh, and it's not every night any more, it's more like once or twice a week. And I do that for dinner. So I'm not really overeating that much. It's when I have the ice cream and sweet stuff later. I don't know, it just feels different.

'What's work in progress? Well, I think I need to do something about feeling angry. I've realised that I am pissed off all the time and that I eat a lot because of that. I've used some of the tools in the feelings tool-kit, but I feel a bit silly bashing a cushion on my own. So I've found a sort of anger-management workshop thingy they're doing near me and I was thinking of going there and seeing what it's like.

'Anything else? Uh, not really. Just to say thanks again to everyone for putting lots of stuff I was thinking into words.'

'Oh am I the last one? Ok. I'm **Olivia**.'

She blushes deeply and bends down to rummage in her bag.

'I've made some notes, but I also wanted to say that it's been incredible to listen to all of you. I don't think I could talk now, if you hadn't all been so honest. Thank you.

'So, what's changed? I've put weight at number one, here. I know it's not about that really, but I lost three stone quite quickly. I just didn't feel like overeating for a while. I did it all really well. I've put a bit back on since then. But not as much as I put back on after dieting. And I'm stable. I've been the same weight for months now. At number two, I've written therapy. When I realised how much my childhood issues impacted my eating, I decided to get some help and I've been seeing a psychotherapist. It's very helpful. The third thing that has changed is that I am training for a 42k women's walk. I'm enjoying it so much although my Gremlin doesn't always make it much fun.

'The second question: "What's work in progress?"
The therapy, obviously and the walk training. And just generally trusting myself and taking my time to get there. I still overeat. But I know I'm doing it, and I don't feel so bad about myself when I do, and the food doesn't work as well most of the time. I'm feeling very hopeful. I don't really have anything else. Just to thank everyone again for being so open.'

'Thank you all so much. It's been really lovely to hear all your stories and the different ways in which you're working with the ideas in the book. I'm so impressed by how much work you've all put into it. It's inspiring. We're going to have a tea break now. We'll see you in half an hour.'

✦

They've all come such a long way . . .

By the time you reach this page, you may be well on your way too. You may have done lots of experimenting and while you know you're not fixed or perfectly sorted, you are hopeful and confident.

And maybe you've done a lot of thinking and you've resisted taking action. We can find every excuse under the sun. Whatever you're doing, right now, it's the best you can.

Take your time. Some of us approach change by thinking about it a lot before we have a go and experiment. And know that reading every book you can get your hands on, going on every course, buying things, none of that will ever change anything. When you are ready . . . *take action.* Experiment. That's the only way to make changes. You don't have to change every-thing all in one go (in fact, as you know by now, it's far better not to). It takes willingness and effort. And it's do-able. All of it.

The route to balance and freedom doesn't follow a nice straight line – it's more like a spiral. Round and round, onwards and upwards. And always, we revisit the same issues, the same problems, the same fears. Nothing changes and everything changes. Round and round. On and on. The aim is not to reach the end – there is no end; the aim is to keep moving, keep learn-ing, keep feeling, keep thinking, keep discovering.

So when you're ready, take a risk, a small one, the smallest one you can think of. Have a go. However difficult, impossible, exciting, crazy or scary it feels, you won't regret it. What lies beyond . . . is freedom.

Welcome to your life Beyond Temptation.

Log On for More

I**T DOESN'T ALL END HERE**. Reading this book is a starting point. There are many ways to support yourself as you go Beyond Temptation, and we'd love to be part of your journey.

DOWNLOAD THE BEYOND TEMPTATION SUPPORT PACK

The Support Pack is crammed full of goodies including:

✦ audio downloads (mp3), which you can listen to again and again for inspiration and guidance

✦ action checklists you can customise and print off

✦ a very practical, pocket-sized guide to tuning in, which you can whip out whenever and wherever you may need it

✦ a suggested reading list with books we've found useful over the years (and which expand on some of the themes in this book)

✦ and a few other surprises, log on to find out what they are . . .

The Beyond Temptation Support Pack is FREE and only a click away. Download it now at www.beyondchocolate.co.uk. Consider it a bonus secret superpower!

JOIN THE FORUM

Would you like to meet and get support from women like Alice, Becky, Christine and all the other wonderful characters in this book?

The Beyond Chocolate Forum is a welcoming and thriving community of women who have decided to ditch the diets and stop overeating using the Beyond Chocolate and Beyond Temptation approaches.

Access to the forum is completely FREE for one month and, if you decide to stay, you will be asked for a small yearly contribution. This is to ensure that members are all genuinely interested and in good faith, and is used to keep this invaluable resource safe and supportive. You won't ever get anyone trying to sell you stuff or – heaven forbid – trying to rope you into dieting.

BEYOND CHOCOLATE FRIENDLY PROFESSIONALS

You will find a list of Beyond Chocolate friendly professionals on our website: psychotherapists, counsellors, nutritionists, doctors, fitness professionals, coaches, etc., who have completed a Beyond Chocolate for Professionals training course. You can see them, confident in the knowledge that they will understand what you are doing and that they will not suggest you go on a diet or focus solely on your weight as the issue.

About
Beyond Chocolate

THE COMPANY

BEYOND CHOCOLATE, as well as being the title of our first book, is the name of our company. We are an organisation dedicated to empowering women to feel good about the way they eat and they way they look. On our website www. beyondchocolate.co.uk you'll find workbooks, audio (mp3) downloads, online ecourses with email support (from a real person), workshops and retreats. We train professionals (doctors, counsellors, psychotherapists, nutritionists, dieticians, etc.) who want to offer their clients an effective, viable alternative to dieting. We also train Chocolate Fairies. Chocolate Fairies? That's what we call the women who run our workshops and groups. They are ordinary women, like you, like us, who have struggled with overeating and/or weight loss and who know what it's like.

THE BOOK

Our first book *Beyond Chocolate: How to stop yo-yo dieting and lose weight for good* offers a radically different approach to weight loss and body confidence.

THE PRINCIPLES

Beyond Chocolate is based on ten principles. They are not rules or guidelines, they are not imperatives, they are simple, commonsense suggestions which you can experiment with and weave into your daily life in any way that works for you. These ten principles will enhance, improve, support and, ultimately, transform the way you eat and the way you feel about your body. You can experiment with them alongside any of the ideas in this book; *Beyond Chocolate* and *Beyond Temptation* complement each other very well – they are prefect companions.

Tune in

You know this one already!

Eat when you're hungry

By working on your overeating, you're halfway there. And while stopping *over*eating is important for a healthy relationship with food, it's equally important to make sure we do eat when we *are* hungry.

After so many years of dieting and deprivation, hunger can become attractive. Feeling those gnawing pangs in our bellies can bring up thoughts of success and weight loss. If we just wait a little longer . . . if we get through this hunger without eating

. . . will that speed the weight loss up a little? It can be such a lure. Eating when we're hungry is how we start to take care of ourselves. It's how we regain balance and normality.

Do you know when you're hungry? Do you know how you get from ravenous to stuffed? How do you decide when you eat breakfast lunch and dinner? What rules do you have for yourself about when to eat and how do they relate to your body's physiological hunger?

Eat whatever you want

We've already talked about how depriving ourselves is linked with overeating. And eating what you want is about so much more. Eating what you want opens the door to enjoying food, to a healthier, more varied diet. Eating what you want means that you begin to take charge, to ask questions, to find out what you *want* to eat, rather than what you think you *should* or *shouldn't* eat. Eating what you want puts an end to diets, rules and restrictions for ever. Eating what you want is radical, it's liberating and it's empowering.

Put it on a plate, sit down and focus

When eating is not the *main* activity, when we eat in front of the telly, at the computer, on the go . . . when we stand in the kitchen and pick at a bit of this or a bit of that . . . when we rush a meal or get so involved in a good conversation that we don't notice what we are eating . . . we miss the experience of eating! Sometimes that's the goal. And now that you are exploring how you overeat, how you use food as a distraction or to manage your life, this principle can help to bring your attention to the food you choose to eat.

When you put it on a plate, sit down and focus on the food, your experience of eating will be radically different. You'll taste it like you've never tasted it before. And if you are over-eating and you are really not hungry at all, that will be so clear, so obvious. When it's just you and the food, there's nowhere to hide.

Stop when you're satisfied

Do you know the difference between being *full* and being *satisfied*? Have you ever eaten a whole meal and still fancied something . . . not felt quite finished?

Being satisfied means we are ready to stop. We have had enough and are happy to stop eating. Satisfaction depends on eating what you want; it depends on being hungry to start with and paying attention to the food you're eating. Recognising how much is *enough* – how much you need to feel happy to stop – is not the same as stopping when you are full. Slowing down and tuning in will help you recognise satisfaction.

Enjoy!

We spend so much time worrying about food, feeling guilty about what we have eaten, eating things we don't particularly like, torturing ourselves about the size of our thighs, pushing ourselves into exercise routines that we don't enjoy . . .

It's time to bring back pleasure, excitement, enjoyment. When we eat what we enjoy and move for pleasure it completely transforms our experience and, apart from being patently more pleasant, we also have a built-in motivator. It's not hard do something we love; it's not a struggle to keep going when we enjoy the process.

Own your body

Owning your body is the starting point for feeling good about the way you look, and weight loss, if that's what you want. We cannot change what we refuse to own.

Owning your body means treating it with respect and kindness, even if you hate it. Owning your body means getting to know it; it means not ignoring it or treating it like a *thing*, an object to be moulded, changed, criticised or judged. You can own your body by wearing clothes that are the right size for you, that fit you well. You can own your body by silencing the Gremlin which constantly tells you that you are too fat and is nasty about the way you look, or by stopping the morning weigh-ins and the punishing exercise regimes. You can own your body by listening to it, paying attention to it.

You don't have to like your body or accept it to own it; you just need to begin to treat yourself – your body – with kindness and respect. Owning your body is a powerful and life-changing principle.

Move!

Moving is vital for good health. Not exercise, MOVING. We can live healthy lives without the gym, organised sport or dance classes. We all just need to MOVE. To use our bodies. To do something physical. If you enjoy any of the aforementioned, that's fine – there's nothing wrong with them at all, so keep doing them, do more of them, if you feel like it. The key is to *move* and whatever you choose to do to get your muscles working, choose something you like doing. Even better, choose something you love doing. Something that brings a flush to your cheeks and a smile to your lips. Do it because you enjoy it, not because it's going to make you lose weight or tone up. And if there's nothing that you enjoy, if you'd rather stay indoors and read a good book any day, or if the idea of moving is simply groan inducing, then consider finding ways to incorporate more movement into your everyday life, rather than making it a separate activity. Or, take yourself gently by the hand and go for a walk. A short one to start with. Put your shoes on and go. Start by walking round the block, and promise yourself that if by the time you reach the end of the road you really hate it, you will go home. The important thing is to make a start.

Whether you enjoy walking, running, swimming, salsa, tennis, netball, football, step, the treadmill, spinning, five rhythms, yoga, Pilates, all of them or none of them, you don't have to get hooked into the all-or-nothing trap. You don't *have* to do it three times a week for the rest of your life. You don't have to exercise at all, you just have to MOVE. Plan to do whatever you like ONCE and then, when you've done it, if you enjoyed it, decide when you'll do it again. One day at a time.

Support yourself

Thinking that strong women, capable women can manage alone, or that they don't need to ask for help, is pretty much the opposite of the way we see it.

Finding ways to support ourselves is the only way to make changes. Knowing when we need to reach out to people who can support, encourage and guide us is a strength, not a weakness. And developing helpful self-supporting strategies and habits means we'll keep going, we won't give up at the first, second or third hurdle. When the going gets tough (as they say.) reach out and ask for some help. Ask someone who knows how to support you and, if they don't know, let them know what works for you, let them know *how* to support you, and practise receiving.

Be your own guru

Beyond Chocolate is not a system, it's not a programme or a method (and neither is Beyond Temptation), and, as you know only too well by now, it's certainly not a diet (in any shape or form) or a lifestyle change.

Our aim is to offer you some ideas to experiment with, some tools to have a go with, some questions to ask yourself. You know yourself better than anyone else. You have all the answers, even though it may not feel like it. Being your own guru is about trusting yourself. Right now, you may feel a million miles away from that. It's so glib to just say, 'Trust yourself'. For many of us, one of the main reasons we are where we are with food is that we *don't* trust ourselves. How can we when we see what we've let ourselves do, what we have allowed ourselves to become?

Our goal is to guide you to trusting yourself, to being your own guru, slowly but surely. You decide what works and what doesn't – not because we tell you or because it sounds plausible or sensible, but because you have experimented, experienced it for yourself and you *know* whether it works for you or not. The key is to keep coming back to yourself, without comparing your experience to anyone else's. That's how we learn to trust ourselves, how we become our own gurus, by being willing to be curious, to experiment, to make mistakes and mess up, to keep going anyway and keep asking questions, keep taking action and keep making choices. It's messy, it's imperfect, it can be slow, but it works.

WORK WITH SOPHIE

Working though this book and beginning to look at the reasons that fuel our overeating can bring up all sorts of issues and questions and sometimes we don't know how to untangle and make sense these on our own. If you'd like to explore these, in confidence, with someone who has both the experience and the training to guide and support you, Sophie is available for individual sessions either in person, on the phone or on Skype.

Here's what a few of Sophie's clients wrote about their sessions with her:

'Sophie was supportive, gentle and challenging all in helpful proportion' SL

'Sophie's kind, gentle way and fabulous sense of humour made my first ever experience of psychotherapy a motivational and inspirational experience' RC

'Sophie is a warm, curious, encouraging, patient, friendly and engaging therapist. I loved our sessions, every single one, tears and all' SV

'Sophie was always there to guide me through a process that allowed me to reach my own conclusions and decisions. She provided a safe environment to work with the issues that matter to me' HB

If you like the sound of working with Sophie, she is always happy to have a chat on the phone to answer any questions. Take a look at Sophie's page on our website for more information on how to get in touch with her.

COOK WITH AUDREY

Many overeaters and serial dieters have a love/hate approach to cooking. When we stop overeating and start to have a balanced, healthy relationship with food, cooking can become one of life's great pleasures. Being confident in the kitchen, knowing how to take a few fresh ingredients and turn them into a deliciously wholesome meal makes eating so much more satisfying. And when we get up from the table satisfied we are less likely to rummage around in the kitchen cupboards later in search of something 'nice'.

Audrey, also known as The Kitchen Fairy, is passionate about showing people how easy it is to turn out simple, tasty, home cooked meals without spending hours shopping or slaving away at the stove. The Kitchen Fairy will teach you the tricks of basic menu planning and how to cook a handful of simple dishes that you love and will want to make over and over again. You won't only be eating well, you'll also be saving money by wasting less food and relying less on overpriced, overprocessed food.

If you would like arrange a Cook Session with Audrey you can find out more on her page on our website and get started with a free weekly menu plan.

✦

To find out more about Beyond Chocolate or, if you have any questions about anything you've read in this book, we'd love to hear from you. Visit www.beyondchocolate.co.uk or drop us a line us any time at info@beyondchocolate.co.uk.

Index

A Benjamin Blog
and His Inquisitive Dog
Guide

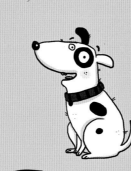

India

Anita Ganeri

Raintree is an imprint of Capstone Global Library Limited, a company incorporated in England and Wales having its registered office at 7 Pilgrim Street, London, EC4V 6LB – Registered company number: 6695582

www.raintreepublishers.co.uk
myorders@raintreepublishers.co.uk

Edited by Dan Nunn, Helen Cox Cannons, and Gina Kammer
Designed by Jo Hinton-Malivoire
Picture research by Ruth Blair and Hannah Taylor
Production by Helen McCreath
Originated by Capstone Global Library Ltd
Printed and bound in Dubai by Oriental Press

ISBN 978 1 406 28105 7 (hardback)
18 17 16 15 14
10 9 8 7 6 5 4 3 2 1

ISBN 978 1 406 28114 9 (paperback)
19 18 17 16 15
10 9 8 7 6 5 4 3 2 1

British Library Cataloguing in Publication Data
A full catalogue record for this book is available from the British Library.

Acknowledgements
We would like to thank the following for permission to reproduce photographs:

Alamy: brianindia, 17, Paul Prescott, 15, Stephen Ford, 14, Stuart Forster, 24, szefei wong, 12, Thomas Cockrem, 22, travelib history, 7, Universal Images Group Ltd., 11; Corbis: ZUMA Press/Prasanta Biswas, 27; Getty Images: Amar Grover, 18, Ben Edwards, 13, Danita Delimont, 10, DreamPictures, 23, Joao Figueiredo, 6, Kurt Werby, 4, Martin Child, 16, Martin Harvey, 8, Subir Basak, 19; Shutterstock: Globe Turner, 28, Mazzzur, cover, Rajesh Narayanan, 25, saiko3p, 26, 29; Superstock: Steve Vidler, 20, Stock Connection, 9, 21

Every effort has been made to contact copyright holders of material reproduced in this book. Any omissions will be rectified in subsequent printings if notice is given to the publisher.

Some words are shown in bold, **like this**. You can find out what they mean by looking in the glossary.

Contents

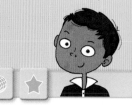

Welcome to India!

Hello! My name is Benjamin Blog and this is Barko Polo, my **inquisitive** dog. (He is named after ancient ace explorer, **Marco Polo**.) We have just got back from our latest adventure – exploring India. We put this book together from some of the blog posts we wrote on the way.

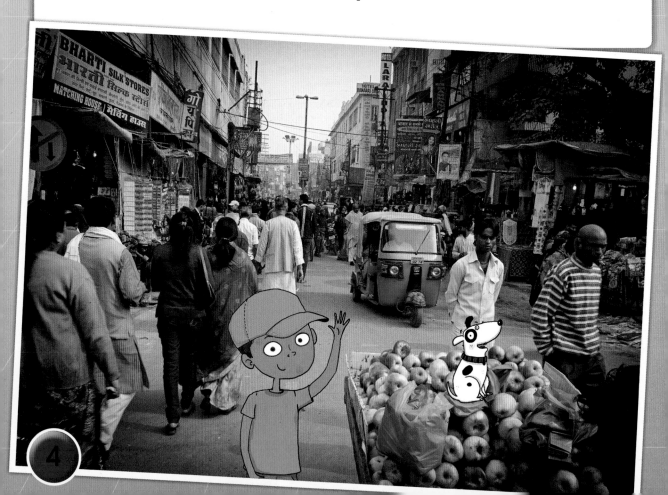

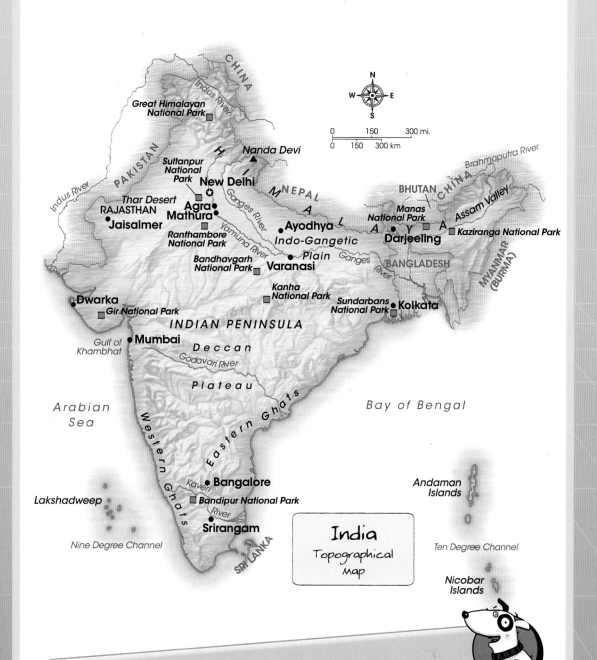

India
Topographical Map

BARKO'S BLOG-TASTIC INDIA FACTS

India is a huge country in South Asia. It is shaped a bit like a triangle with the Arabian Sea on one side, the Bay of Bengal on the other, and the Himalayas across the top.

Historic places

Posted by: Ben Blog | 4 December at 10.00 a.m.

We started our tour at Fatehpur Sikri, the ancient capital city built by the **Mughal emperor** Akbar. He ruled India about 450 years ago. Nobody lives here now, but you can wander around the beautiful palaces and have your picture taken next to the grave of Akbar's favourite elephant.

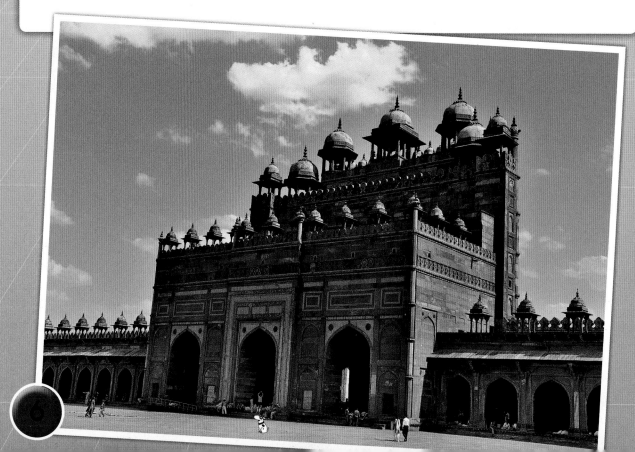

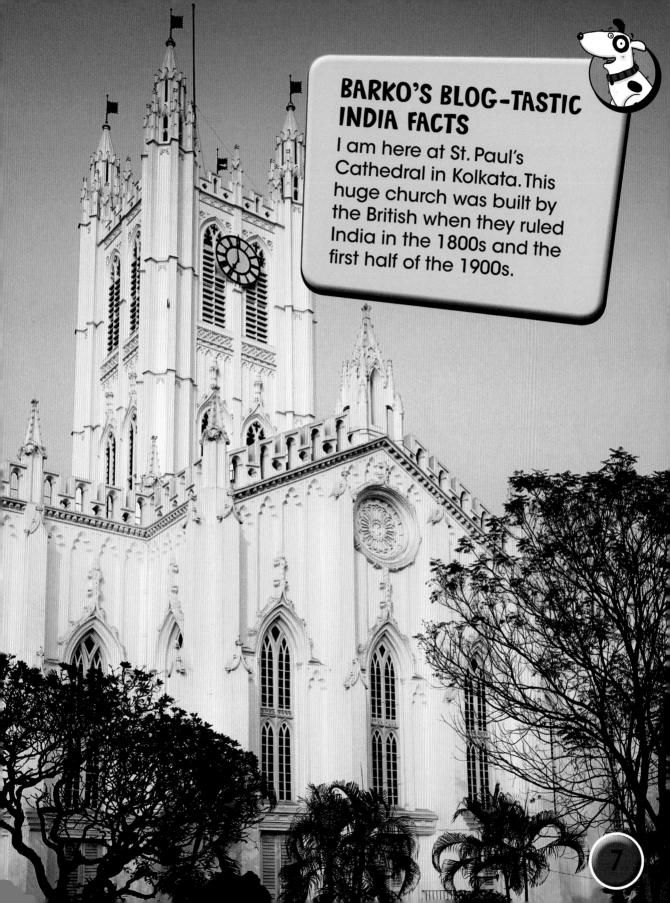

BARKO'S BLOG-TASTIC INDIA FACTS

I am here at St. Paul's Cathedral in Kolkata. This huge church was built by the British when they ruled India in the 1800s and the first half of the 1900s.

Rivers, mountains, and deserts

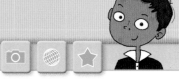

Posted by: Ben Blog | 18 December at 2.10 p.m.

From Fatehpur Sikri, we caught the train to Varanasi on the banks of the river Ganges. The river flows from the Himalayas, across India, and into the Bay of Bengal. For **Hindus**, it is a holy river. They believe that bathing in the water will wash away any bad things they have done.

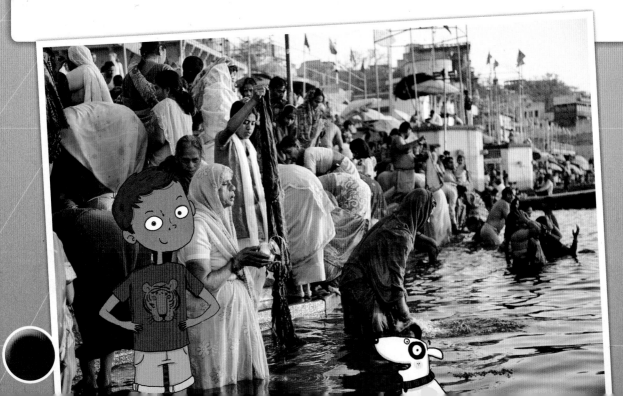

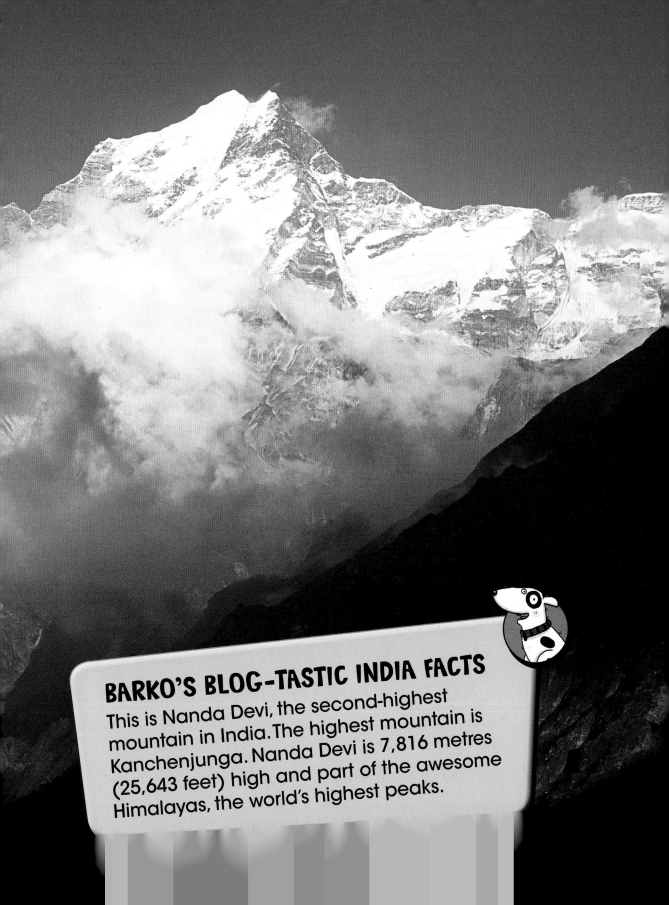

BARKO'S BLOG-TASTIC INDIA FACTS

This is Nanda Devi, the second-highest mountain in India. The highest mountain is Kanchenjunga. Nanda Devi is 7,816 metres (25,643 feet) high and part of the awesome Himalayas, the world's highest peaks.

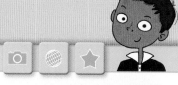

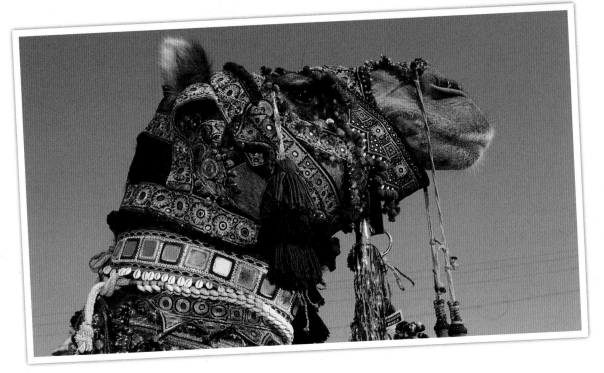

Our next stop was the dusty Thar Desert, where we arrived just in time for the camel festival. It lasts for five days, and people come from all over the desert to buy and sell their camels. There is even a "best-dressed camel" contest. Here is a photo I took of this year's winner.

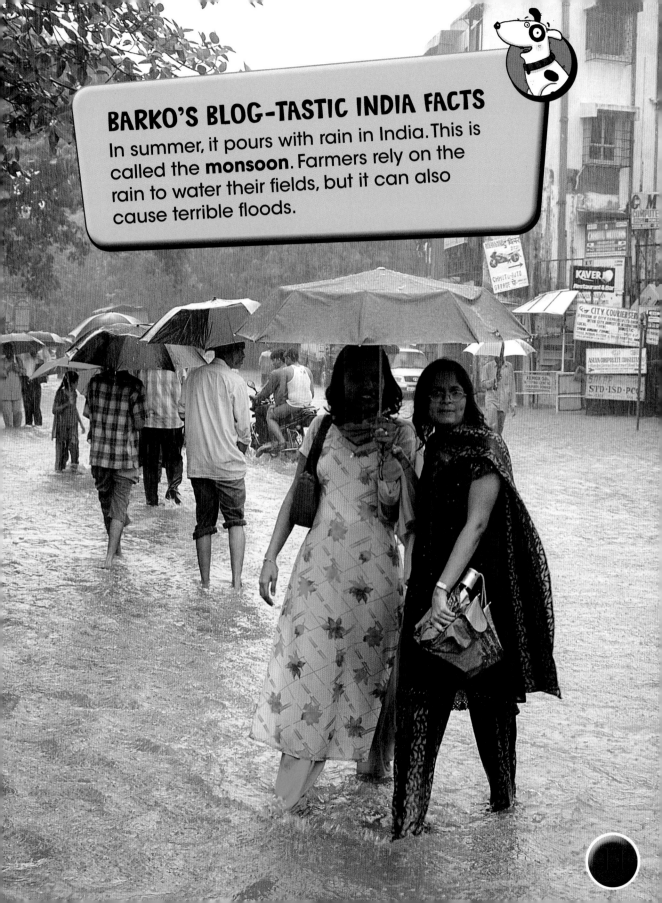

BARKO'S BLOG-TASTIC INDIA FACTS

In summer, it pours with rain in India. This is called the **monsoon**. Farmers rely on the rain to water their fields, but it can also cause terrible floods.

Crowded cities

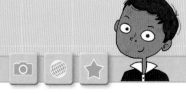

Posted by: Ben Blog | 30 March at 4.36 p.m.

This morning we arrived in New Delhi, India's capital city. What a busy, bustling place. We hitched a ride on a **rickshaw** to the Red Fort in the old part of the city. Like Fatehpur Sikri, the Red Fort was built by the **Mughals**, and it gets its name from its massive red **sandstone** walls.

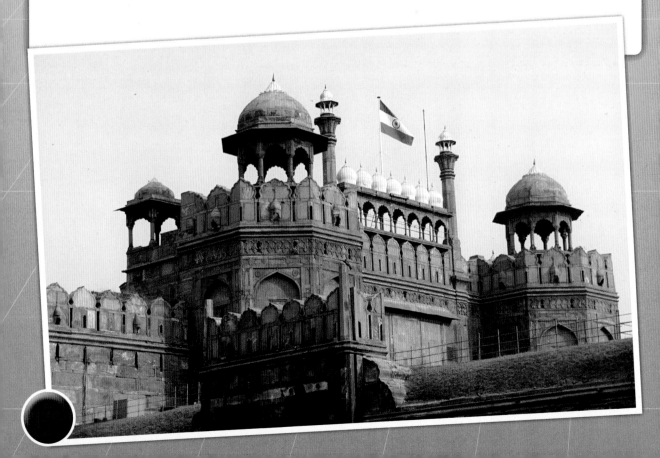

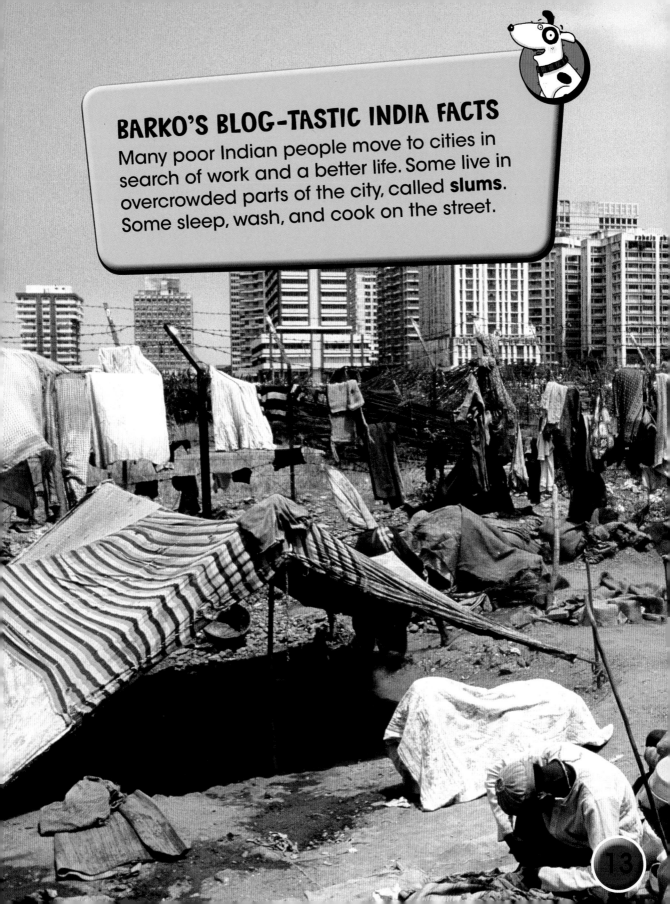

BARKO'S BLOG-TASTIC INDIA FACTS
Many poor Indian people move to cities in search of work and a better life. Some live in overcrowded parts of the city, called **slums**. Some sleep, wash, and cook on the street.

Namaste!

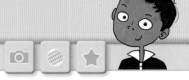

Namaste means "hello" in Hindi. When you say *namaste*, you put your hands together and bow your head. Hindi is the most commonly spoken language in India, especially here in the north. But there are 21 other main languages and many local **dialects** to learn.

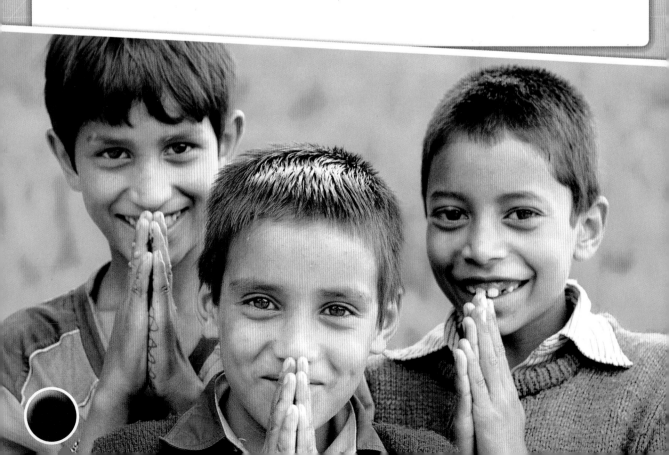

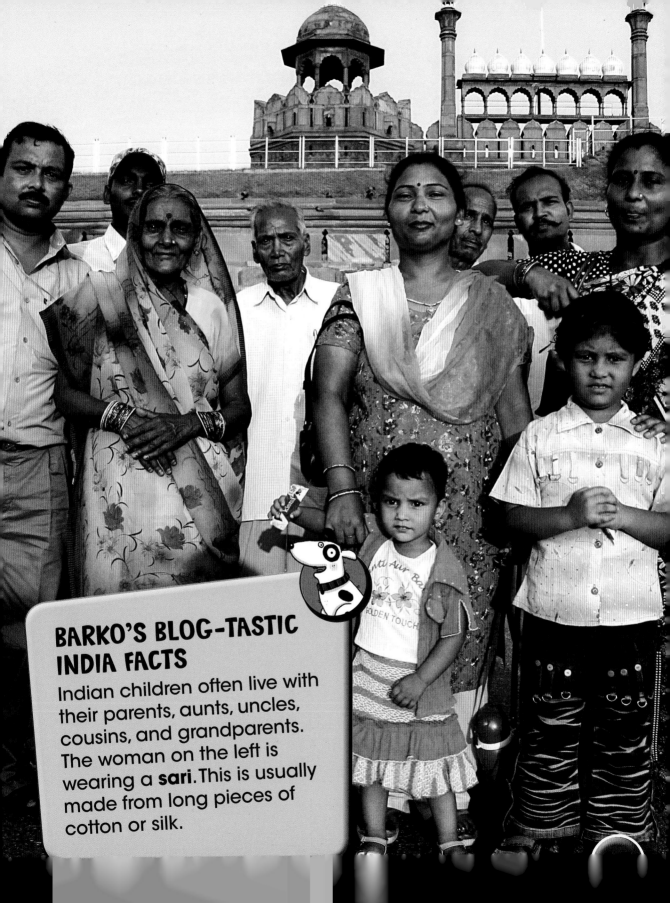

BARKO'S BLOG-TASTIC INDIA FACTS

Indian children often live with their parents, aunts, uncles, cousins, and grandparents. The woman on the left is wearing a **sari**. This is usually made from long pieces of cotton or silk.

In the big cities, many people live in large blocks of apartments. But, a short bus ride out of the city, and we are in the countryside. Most Indian people live in small villages and work by farming the land. They live in small, simple houses with their animals outside.

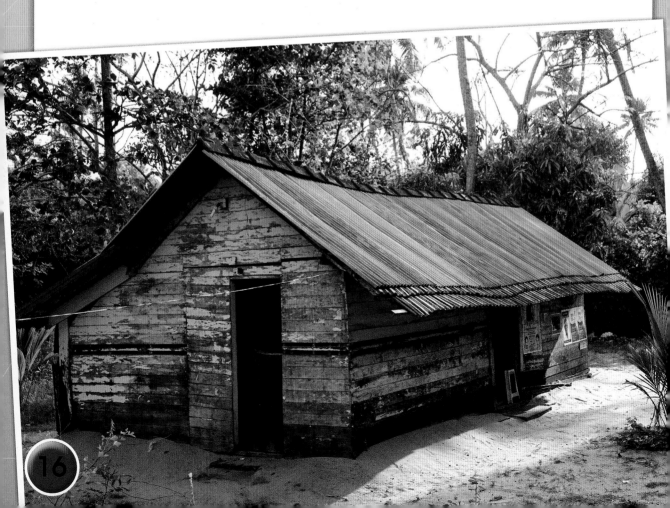

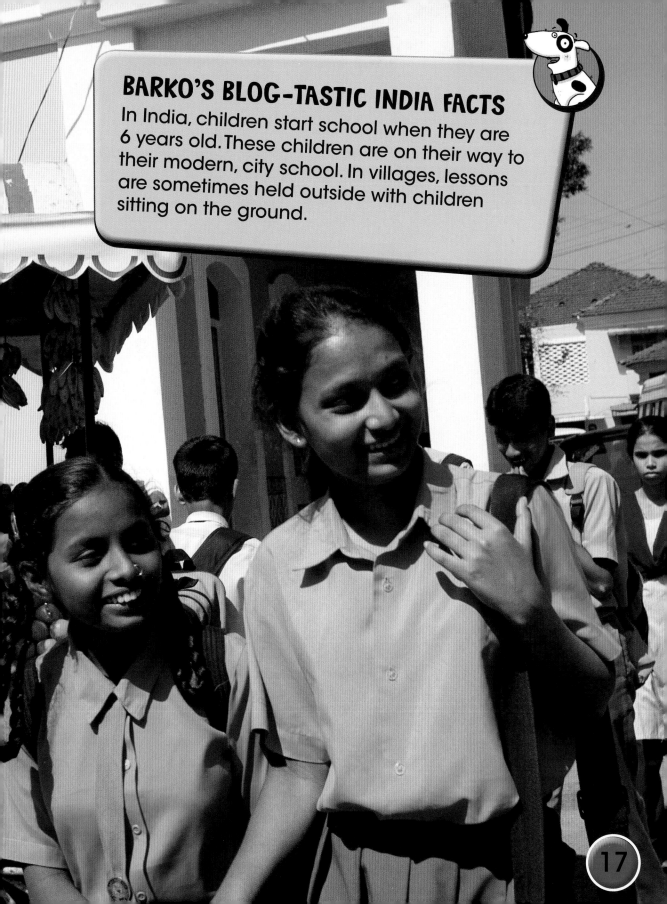

BARKO'S BLOG-TASTIC INDIA FACTS

In India, children start school when they are 6 years old. These children are on their way to their modern, city school. In villages, lessons are sometimes held outside with children sitting on the ground.

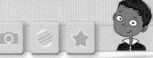

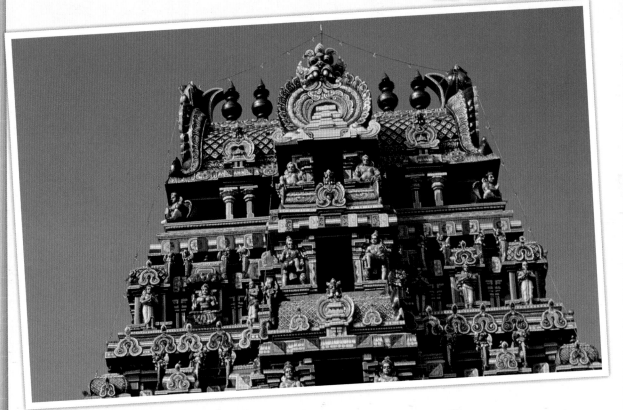

We have travelled south to Tamil Nadu. It is famous for its temples, such as this one at Srirangam. Most Indians are **Hindus**, who follow the religion of **Hinduism**. A temple is a place where they worship. This stunning tower is the gateway to the temple and is covered in carvings of the Hindu gods and goddesses.

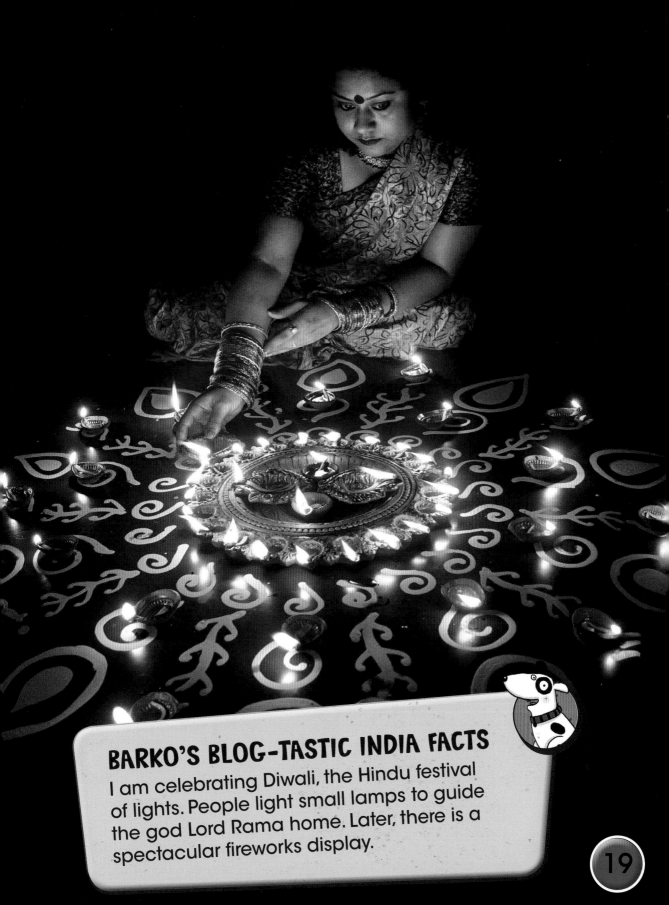

BARKO'S BLOG-TASTIC INDIA FACTS

I am celebrating Diwali, the Hindu festival of lights. People light small lamps to guide the god Lord Rama home. Later, there is a spectacular fireworks display.

Feeling hungry?

Posted by: Ben Blog | 3 November at 6.10 p.m.

All this travelling makes Barko and me hungry, so we stopped for an Indian meal. Most Hindus are vegetarians and do not eat meat. They like to eat spicy vegetables with rice or flatbreads. Here in the south, crispy rice pancakes, called dosas, are very popular. Yummy!

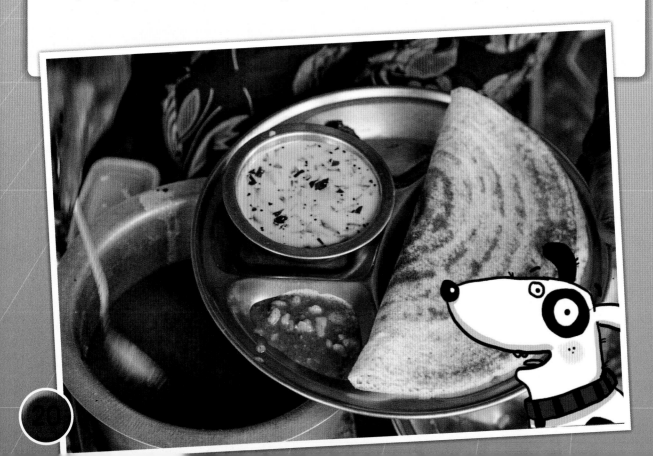

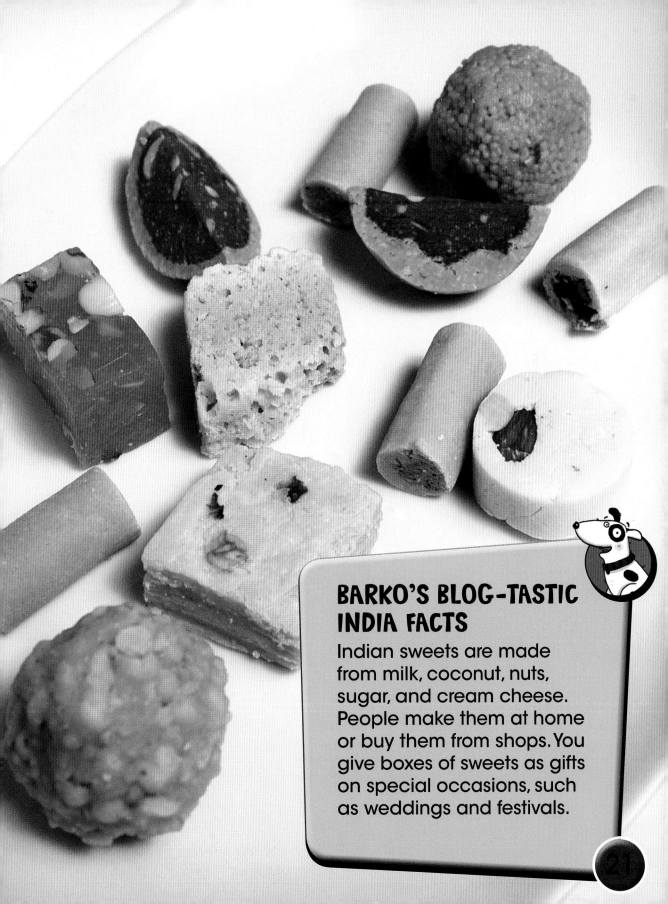

BARKO'S BLOG-TASTIC INDIA FACTS

Indian sweets are made from milk, coconut, nuts, sugar, and cream cheese. People make them at home or buy them from shops. You give boxes of sweets as gifts on special occasions, such as weddings and festivals.

21

Fun and games

Posted by: Ben Blog | 11 December at 3.32 p.m.

Next, we flew east to the city of Kolkata to watch a cricket match. Indians are crazy about cricket and play in the street, on the beach, or in the park – wherever they can find space. Members of the Indian cricket team are national heroes. When they are playing, the city comes to a stop.

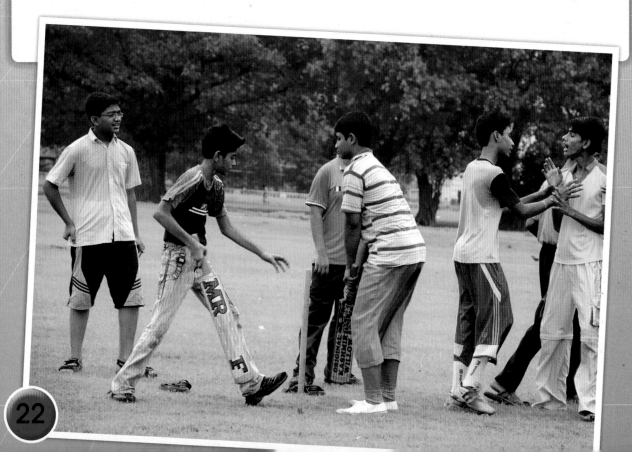

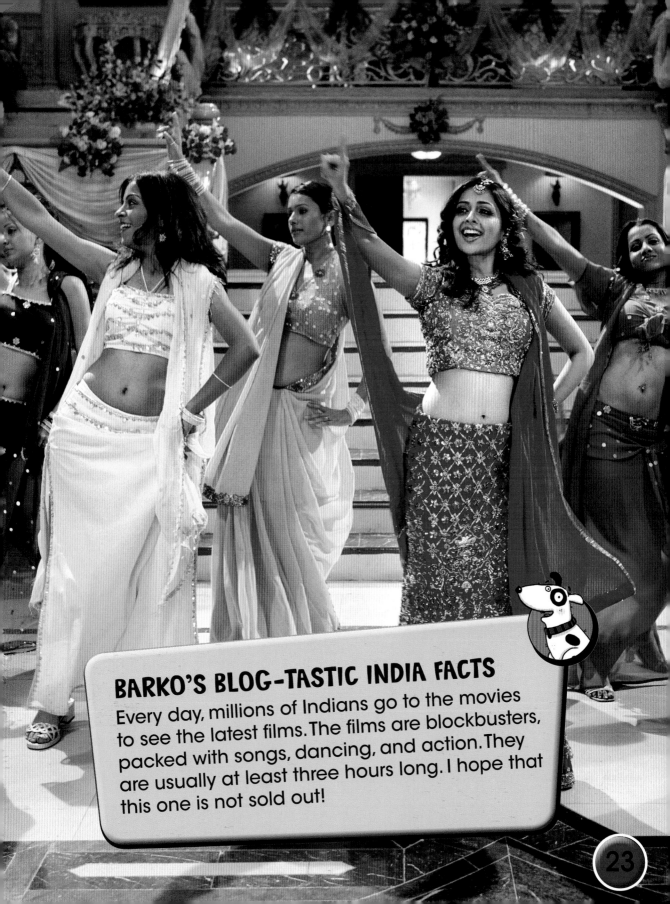

BARKO'S BLOG-TASTIC INDIA FACTS

Every day, millions of Indians go to the movies to see the latest films. The films are blockbusters, packed with songs, dancing, and action. They are usually at least three hours long. I hope that this one is not sold out!

From TVs to tea leaves

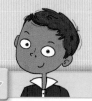

Posted by: Ben Blog | 28 December at 8.23 a.m.

My laptop wasn't working properly, and I needed to get it fixed. So, we headed to Bangalore, India's centre for IT (information technology). Thousands of people work with computers here. Factories in India also make TVs, washing machines, and cars. This has made some Indians very rich, but millions of people are still desperately poor.

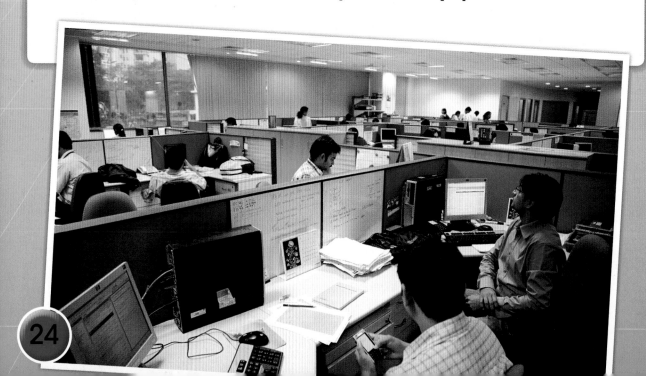

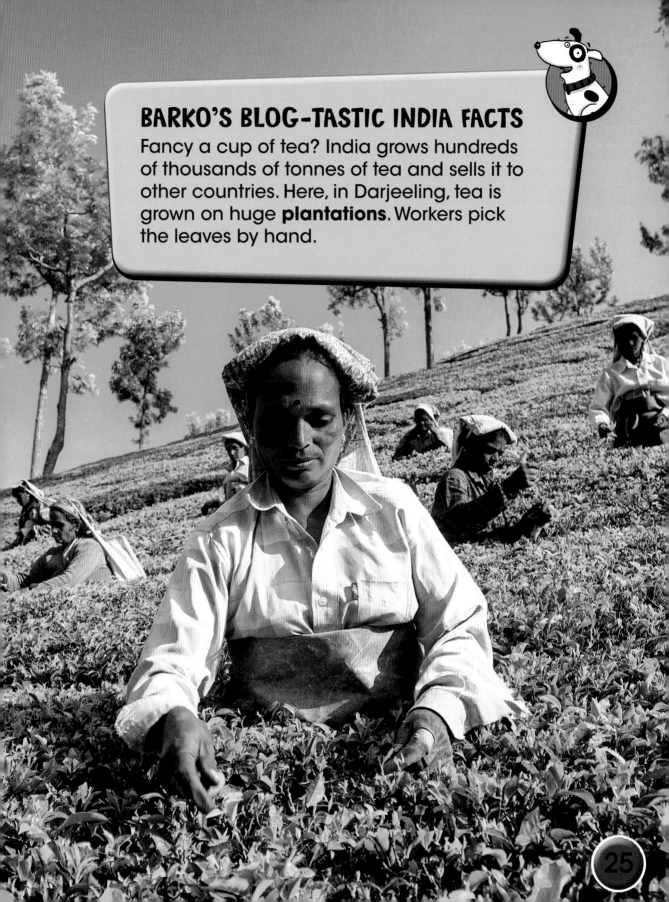

BARKO'S BLOG-TASTIC INDIA FACTS

Fancy a cup of tea? India grows hundreds of thousands of tonnes of tea and sells it to other countries. Here, in Darjeeling, tea is grown on huge **plantations**. Workers pick the leaves by hand.

And finally ...

Our trip is nearly over, and we have saved the best for last. We are here in Agra to see the Taj Mahal. It is one of the world's most famous buildings, so I took loads of pictures. It was built in the 1600s by **Mughal emperor** Shah Jahan in memory of his dead wife. What a sight!

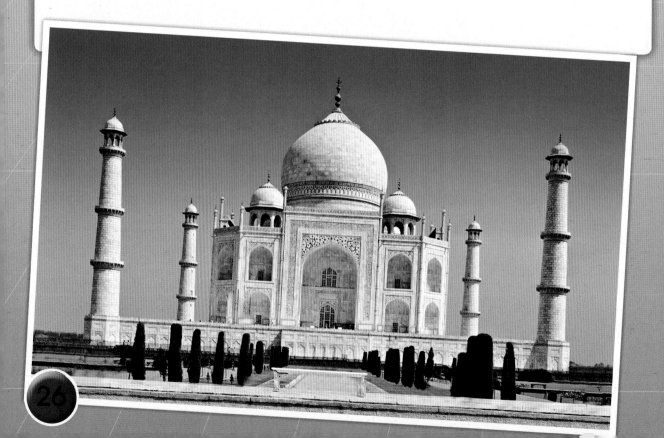

26

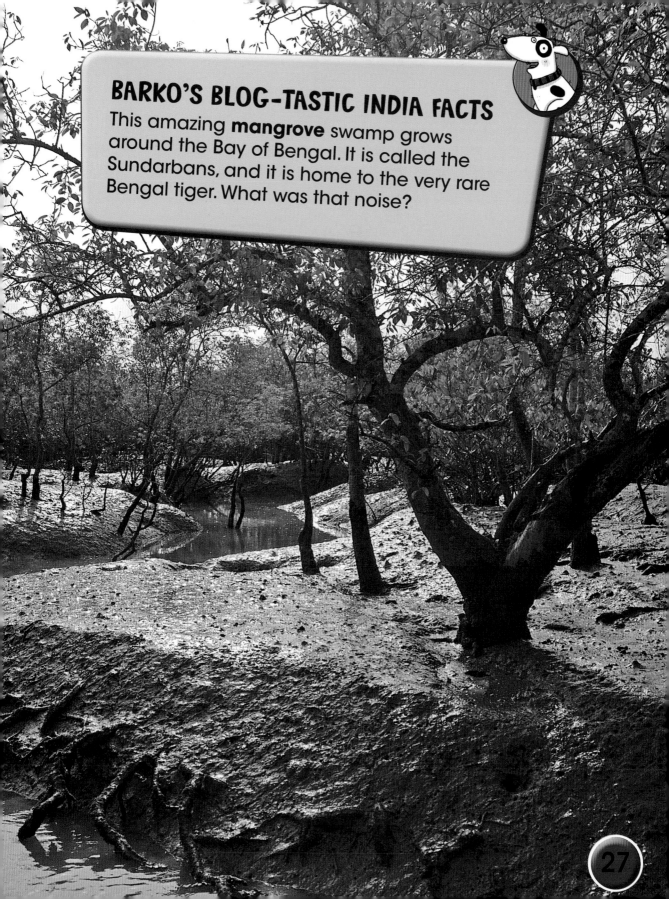

BARKO'S BLOG-TASTIC INDIA FACTS

This amazing **mangrove** swamp grows around the Bay of Bengal. It is called the Sundarbans, and it is home to the very rare Bengal tiger. What was that noise?

India fact file

Area: 3,288,000 square kilometres
(1,269,500 square miles)

Population: 1,220,800,000 (2013)

Capital city: New Delhi

Other main cities: Mumbai; Kolkata

Languages: Hindi and 21 other official languages

Main religions: **Hinduism**; Islam;
Christianity; Sikhism

Highest mountain: Kanchenjunga
(8,598 metres/28,209 feet)

Longest river: Brahmaputra
(2,840 kilometres/1,764 miles)

Currency: Indian rupee

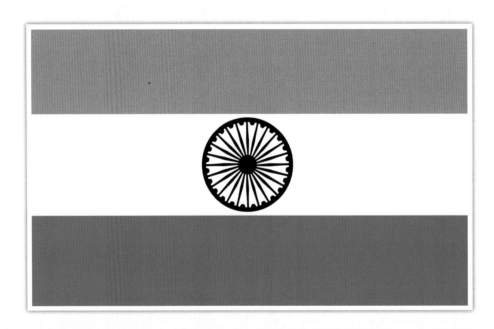

India quiz

Find out how much you know about India with our quick quiz.

1. What is a **sari**?
a) an Indian sweet
b) an Indian piece of clothing
c) an Indian musical instrument

2. What does *namaste* mean?
a) hello
b) good-bye
c) how are you?

3. Where do **Hindus** worship?
a) in a mosque
b) in a church
c) in a temple

4. Which is the most popular sport in India?
a) football
b) kite-flying
c) cricket

5. What is this?

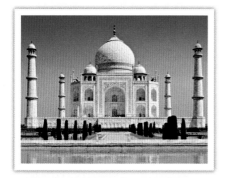

Answers
1. b
2. a
3. c
4. c
5. Taj Mahal

Glossary

dialect a language spoken in a small area or by a small number of people

emperor a ruler

Hindu a person who follows the Hinduism religion

Hinduism an Indian religion, followed by Hindus

inquisitive being interested in learning about the world

mangrove a tree that grows along some tropical coasts

Marco Polo an explorer who lived from about 1254 to 1324; he travelled from Italy to China

monsoon a wind that brings heavy rain

Mughal people who ruled India from the 1500s to the 1800s

plantation a large farm where crops, such as tea and bananas, are grown

rickshaw a small vehicle for carrying passengers, often pulled by a man on a bicycle

sandstone a soft, reddish rock

sari a long piece of cloth that is wrapped around a woman's body

slum an overcrowded part of a city where poor people live

Find out more

Books

India. (Countries Around the World), Ali Brownlie Bojang (Raintree, 2012)

India (My Country), Jillian Powell (Franklin Watts, 2013)

We Visit India (Your Land and My Land), Khadija Ejaz (Mitchell Lane Publishers, 2014)

Websites

kids.nationalgeographic.com/kids/places
The National Geographic website has lots of information, photos, and maps of countries around the world.

www.worldatlas.com
Packed with information about various countries, this website includes flags, time zones, facts, maps, and timelines.

Index